Robert Salmon, DSW
Roberta Graziano, DSW
Editors

Group Work and Aging: Issues in Practice, Research, and Education

Group Work and Aging: Issues in Practice, Research, and Education has been co-published simultaneously as *Journal of Gerontological Social Work*, Volume 44, Numbers 1/2 2004.

Pre-publication
REVIEWS,
COMMENTARIES,
EVALUATIONS . . .

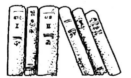

"Salmon and Graziano take us on the 'Grand Tour' of group work with the aged. From the struggles of the beginning worker influenced by societal and professional stereotypes of the aged, to approaches by savvy, experienced group workers, we are gifted with CASE-AUGMENTED ART-ICLES THAT ILLUSTRATE GROUP WORK PRACTICE AT ITS FINEST. Chapter subjects include telephone groups, support groups with care-givers, immigrants, aged parents of mentally ill persons, terminally ill aged, and an intergenerational sing-ing group highlighting the use of pro-gram activities."

Paul Abels, PhD, MSW
President
Association for the Advancement
of Social Work with Groups (AASWG)
Professor Emeritus
Department of Social Work
California State University
Long Beach

More pre-publication
REVIEWS, COMMENTARIES, EVALUATIONS . . .

"MANDATORY READING for practitioners who work with older adults, for any course that focuses on work with this population, and for field supervisors of social work interns. This is a wonderful, touching, and highly informative collection of chapters ranging from the very personal to high-level scholarship. While this is not a 'how-to' book, it OFFERS MANY POWERFUL EXAMPLES for applying important social group work theories to work with older adults in a variety of contexts by identifying both problems and opportunities."

Dominique Moyse Steinberg, DSW Fellow, ACSW
Director and Founder.
The Center for the Advancement of Mutual Aid™
Author of The Mutual Aid Approach to Working with Groups *and* The Social Work Student's Research Handbook.

"If you want to learn what is distinct and unique about working with groups of older people struggling with mental illness, homelessness, immigration, disability, or with substance abuse issues, READ THIS BOOK. If you want to learn about the use of creative services and group methods (e.g., the use of the telephone, music, art, drama, role play), READ THIS BOOK. Each chapter examines how workers take into account the special issues and needs of each population, how these issues and needs influence group member participation and, most importantly, how the worker develops innovative and responsive group work interventions. The editors, Professors Salmon and Graziano, deserve our praise and appreciation for this magnificent book. IT IS A JEWEL."

Alex Gitterman, EdD
Professor of Social Work
University of Connecticut
School of Social Work

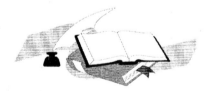

More pre-publication
REVIEWS, COMMENTARIES, EVALUATIONS . . .

"**A** GEM OF A BOOK . . . PUBLISHED AT JUST THE RIGHT TIME! Useful across human service disciplines, this book has much to offer practitioners, administrators, teachers, staff trainers, and those involved with curriculum development. In addition to a great variety of settings included in this book, there are rich descriptions of group services to aging substance abusers, the homeless, persons with mental illness, Asian immigrants and other minority groups, caretakers of adult children with mental illness, lesbians, graduate students, people at the end of life, and home attendants, among others. Readers will learn about up-to-date research findings in aging and group methods; about the special needs of aging persons, their families, and other caregivers; about the everyday activities and struggles of aging persons; about groups of many kinds, including therapy, support, and activity; about the use of technologies; and skills and techniques."

Ralph Dolgoff, DSW
Professor of Social Work
University of Maryland, Baltimore

"**E**DUCATORS, PRACTITIONERS, AND STUDENTS will find this book enormously useful in integrating group methods with practice with the aged. This is integrative work on a high level in which the contributors impart their knowledge about a diverse aging population with examples of how group services have been developed and delivered to the populations they address. As an educator I was delighted to see a chapter devoted to the use of the Record of Service, a practice evaluation instrument which helps students deepen their understanding of their own practice."

Renee Solomon, DSW, LCSW
Associate Professor
Columbia University
School of Social Work (retired)
Consultant, the Fortune Society

Group Work and Aging: Issues in Practice, Research, and Education

Group Work and Aging: Issues in Practice, Research, and Education has been co-published simultaneously as *Journal of Gerontological Social Work*, Volume 44, Numbers 1/2 2004.

Group Work and Aging: Issues in Practice, Research, and Education

Robert Salmon, DSW
Roberta Graziano, DSW
Editors

Group Work and Aging: Issues in Practice, Research, and Education has been co-published simultaneously as *Journal of Gerontological Social Work*, Volume 44, Numbers 1/2 2004.

The Haworth Social Work Practice Press
An Imprint of The Haworth Press, Inc.

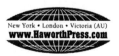

New York • London • Victoria (AU)
www.HaworthPress.com

Published by

The Haworth Social Work Practice Press, 10 Alice Street, Binghamton, NY 13904-1580 USA

The Haworth Social Work Practice Press is an imprint of The Haworth Press, Inc., 10 Alice Street, Binghamton, NY 13904-1580 USA.

Group Work and Aging: Issues in Practice, Research, and Education has been co-published simultaneously as *Journal of Gerontological Social Work,* Volume 44, Numbers 1/2 2004.

The development, preparation, and publication of this work has been undertaken with great care. However, the publisher, employees, editors, and agents of The Haworth Press and all imprints of The Haworth Press, Inc., including The Haworth Medical Press® and Pharmaceutical Products Press®, are not responsible for any errors contained herein or for consequences that may ensue from use of materials or information contained in this work. Opinions expressed by the author(s) are not necessarily those of The Haworth Press, Inc. With regard to case studies, identities and circumstances of individuals discussed herein have been changed to protect confidentiality. Any resemblance to actual persons, living or dead, is entirely coincidental.

Cover design by Marylouise Doyle.

Library of Congress Cataloging-in-Publication Data

Group work and aging: issues in practice, research, and education / Robert Salmon, Roberta Graziano, editors.
     p. cm.
    "Co-published simultaneously as Journal of gerontological social work, volume 44, numbers 1/2 2004."
    Includes bibliographical references and index.
    ISBN-13: 978-0-7890-2880-8 (hc.: alk. paper)
    ISBN-10: 0-7890-2880-8 (hc.: alk. paper)
    ISBN-13: 978-0-7890-2881-5 (pbk.: alk. paper)
    ISBN-10: 0-7890-2881-6 (pbk.: alk. paper)
  1. Social work with older people. 2. Social group work. I. Salmon, Robert, 1930- II. Graziano, Roberta.
III. Journal of gerontological social work.
    HV1451.G75 2004
    362.6-dc22
                                          2004025965

Dignity and Old Age, edited by Rose Dobrof, DSW, and Harry R. Moody, PhD (Vol. 29, No. 2/3, 1998). *"Challenges us to uphold the right to age with dignity, which is embedded in the heart and soul of every man and woman." (H. James Towey, President, Commission on Aging with Dignity, Tallahassee, FL)*

Intergenerational Approaches in Aging: Implications for Education, Policy and Practice, edited by Kevin Brabazon, MPA, and Robert Disch, MA (Vol. 28, No. 1/2/3, 1997). *"Provides a wealth of concrete examples of areas in which intergenerational perspectives and knowledge are needed." (Robert C. Atchley, PhD, Director, Scribbs Gerontology Center, Miami University)*

Social Work Response to the White House Conference on Aging: From Issues to Actions, edited by Constance Corley Saltz, PhD, LCSW (Vol. 27, No. 3, 1997). *"Provides a framework for the discussion of issues relevant to social work values and practice, including productive aging, quality of life, the psychological needs of older persons, and family issues." (Jordan I. Kosberg, PhD, Professor and PhD Program Coordinator, School of Social Work, Florida International University, North Miami, FL)*

Special Aging Populations and Systems Linkages, edited by M. Joanna Mellor, DSW (Vol. 25, No. 1/2, 1996). *"An invaluable tool for anyone working with older persons with special needs." (Irene Gutheil, DSW, Associate Professor, Graduate School of Social Service, Fordham University)*

New Developments in Home Care Services for the Elderly: Innovations in Policy, Program, and Practice, edited by Lenard W. Kaye, DSW (Vol. 24, No. 3/4, 1995). *"An excellent compilation. . . . Especially pertinent to the functions of administrators, supervisors, and case managers in home care. . . . Highly recommended for every home care agency and a must for administrators and middle managers." (Geriatric Nursing Book Review)*

Geriatric Social Work Education, edited by M. Joanna Mellor, DSW, and Renee Solomon, DSW (Vol. 18, No. 3/4, 1992). *"Serves as a foundation upon which educators and fieldwork instructors can build courses that incorporate more aging content." (SciTech Book News)*

Vision and Aging: Issues in Social Work Practice, edited by Nancy D. Weber, MSW (Vol. 17, No. 3/4, 1992). *"For those involved in vision rehabilitation programs, the book provides practical information and should stimulate readers to revise their present programs of care." (Journal of Vision Rehabilitation)*

Health Care of the Aged: Needs, Policies, and Services, edited by Abraham Monk, PhD (Vol. 15, No. 3/4, 1990). *"The chapters reflect firsthand experience and are competent and informative. Readers . . . will find the book rewarding and useful. The text is timely, appropriate, and well-presented." (Health & Social Work)*

Twenty-Five Years of the Life Review: Theoretical and Practical Considerations, edited by Robert Disch, MA (Vol. 12, No. 3/4, 1989). *This practical and thought-provoking book examines the history and concept of the life review.*

Gerontological Social Work: International Perspectives, edited by Merl C. Hokenstad, Jr., PhD, and Katherine A. Kendall, PhD (Vol. 12, No. 1/2, 1988). *"Makes a very useful contribution in examining the changing role of the social work profession in serving the elderly." (Journal of the International Federation on Ageing)*

Gerontological Social Work Practice with Families: A Guide to Practice Issues and Service Delivery, edited by Rose Dobrof, DSW (Vol. 10, No. 1/2, 1987). *An in-depth examination of the importance of family relationships within the context of social work practice with the elderly.*

Ethnicity and Gerontological Social Work, edited by Rose Dobrof, DSW (Vol. 9, No. 4, 1987). *"Addresses the issues of ethnicity with great sensitivity. Most of the topics addressed here are rarely addressed in other literature." (Dr. Milada Disman, Department of Behavioral Science, University of Toronto)*

Social Work and Alzheimer's Disease, edited by Rose Dobrof, DSW (Vol. 9, No. 2, 1986). *"New and innovative social work roles with Alzheimer's victims and their families in both hospital and non-hospital settings." (Continuing Education Update)*

Indexing, Abstracting & Website/Internet Coverage

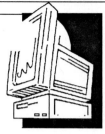

This section provides you with a list of major indexing & abstracting services and other tools for bibliographic access. That is to say, each service began covering this periodical during the year noted in the right column. Most Websites which are listed below have indicated that they will either post, disseminate, compile, archive, cite or alert their own Website users with research-based content from this work. (This list is as current as the copyright date of this publication.)

(continued)

(continued)

(continued)

Special Bibliographic Notes related to special journal issues (separates) and indexing/abstracting:

- indexing/abstracting services in this list will also cover material in any "separate" that is co-published simultaneously with Haworth's special thematic journal issue or DocuSerial. Indexing/abstracting usually covers material at the article/chapter level.
- monographic co-editions are intended for either non-subscribers or libraries which intend to purchase a second copy for their circulating collections.
- monographic co-editions are reported to all jobbers/wholesalers/approval plans. The source journal is listed as the "series" to assist the prevention of duplicate purchasing in the same manner utilized for books-in-series.
- to facilitate user/access services all indexing/abstracting services are encouraged to utilize the co-indexing entry note indicated at the bottom of the first page of each article/chapter/contribution.
- this is intended to assist a library user of any reference tool (whether print, electronic, online, or CD-ROM) to locate the monographic version if the library has purchased this version but not a subscription to the source journal.
- individual articles/chapters in any Haworth publication are also available through the Haworth Document Delivery Service (HDDS).

This volume is for my own mutual aid group:
Sheila, who is always there and a constant source
of inspiration and support, and

| Julie and Glenn | Dena and Jonathan | Laura and Jerald |
| Elizabeth and Gary | Emily and Rachel | Leo |

-Bob Salmon

And for John, Laura, Paul, Will, Franklin, and Anna,
who illuminate and enrich my life every day.

-Roberta Graziano

We thank Mary McGilvray and Esther Rohatiner
for their assistance and efforts in the preparation of this volume.

ABOUT THE EDITORS

Robert Salmon, DSW, is Professor at Hunter College School of Social Work. After joining the faculty in 1971, he later served as Associate Dean or Interim Dean for 16 years. He has been a consulting editor for the *Journal of Gerontological Social Work* for over 20 years, and also serves in this capacity for three other social work journals. He has presented many papers on social group work practice nationally and internationally. He has published many articles on group work practice and other areas such as work with the aging, drug addiction, and issues in social policy. Two books with Roselle Kurland are *Teaching a Methods Course in Social Work with Groups* and *Group Work Practice in a Troubled Society: Problems and Opportunities.* He served on the board of directors of the Association for the Advancement of Social Work with Groups for 12 years, including nine years as treasurer of this international organization. He received the Hunter College Award for Excellence in Teaching in 1998. He has received well over 125 grants for the school, including a number with his friend, colleague, and co-editor of this volume, Roberta Graziano.

Roberta Graziano, DSW, is Professor and currently Interim Associate Dean at Hunter College School of Social Work. She serves as a consulting editor for the *Journal of Gerontological Social Work* and the *Journal of Teaching in Social Work* and was for many years consulting editor for the *Child and Adolescent Social Work Journal.* For nearly 20 years she served in various capacities (including president and program chair) on the board of the International Conference for the Advancement of Private Practice. She has published numerous articles on clinical social work, with particular emphasis on trauma, and has served as co-author of articles on the use of group work by work-study MSW students for older adults and their families. Professor Graziano developed the Aging and Health Work-Study MSW Program at Hunter, the first of its kind, with her co-director, Robert Salmon.

Group Work and Aging: Issues in Practice, Research, and Education

CONTENTS

About the Contributors

Sister Maria Theresa Amato, OP, MSW, is affiliated with Sisters of St. Dominic, Brooklyn, New York.

Irene Chung, PhD, CSW, is Assistant Professor, Hunter College School of Social Work, New York, New York.

Miriam Cusicanqui, MSW, is Coordinator, CAPS Program, Goddard Riverside Community Center, New York, New York.

Kris Drumm, MSW, is Group Work consultant and trainer, Wilton Manors, Florida.

Helene Ebenstein, MSW, is affiliated with The Mount Sinai Medical Center, The Mount Sinai Hospital, New York, New York.

Ann Goelitz, MSW, CSW, is Clinical Social Work Supervisor, Women's Health Project, St. Luke's-Roosevelt Hospital Center, New York, New York.

Harriet Goodman, DSW, is Associate Professor, Hunter College School of Social Work, New York, New York.

Roberta Graziano, DSW, is Professor, and Interim Associate Dean, Hunter College School of Social Work, New York, New York.

Frank Guida, PhD, is Director of Research, Odyssey House, New York, New York.

Timothy B. Kelly, PhD, is Senior Research Fellow, Glasgow Caledonian University School of Nursing, Midwifery, and Community Health, Glasgow, Scotland.

Andrew Malekoff, MSW, is Associate Director, North Shore Child and Family Guidance Center, Roslyn Heights, New York, and Editor, *Social Work with Groups.*

M. Joanna Mellor, DSW, is Visiting Assistant Professor, Wurzweiler School of Social Work, Yeshiva University, New York, New York.

Peter Provet, PhD, is President and CEO, Odyssey House, New York, New York.

Barbara H. Reinhart, PhD, is Field Instructor, Hunter College School of Social Work, New York, New York.

Victoria M. Rizzo, PhD, is Research Assistant Professor and Executive Director, Elder Network of the Capital Region, Institute of Gerontology, School of Social Welfare, University at Albany, State University of New York, Albany, New York.

Robert Salmon, DSW, is Professor, Hunter College School of Social Work, New York, New York.

Tamara L. Smith, is a PhD Candidate, Department of Sociology, and Research Associate, Institute of Gerontology, University of Albany, State University of New York, Albany, New York.

Sarah Stevenson, is an MSW student, Hunter College School of Social Work, New York, New York.

John Tavolacci, MSW, is Senior Vice President, Director of Clinical Services, Odyssey House, New York, New York.

Ronald W. Toseland, PhD, is Professor and Director, Institute of Gerontology, School of Social Welfare, University of Albany, State University of New York, Albany, New York.

Arnold Unterbach, MSW, is Vice President, Director of Mental Health Services, Odyssey House, New York, New York.

Michele A. Zinoman, is a PhD Candidate, School of Social Welfare, University at Albany, State University of New York, Albany, New York.

Foreword

It is with great pleasure that Dr. Dobrof and I present a special volume on group work with older persons to JGSW's readers. Drs. Salmon and Graziano are to be commended for their success in producing this comprehensive and insightful collection. The authors include both well-known leaders in group work practice and those on the brink of their professional careers. Together, they provide a careful look at group work from the macro and micro perspectives.

All social workers, whatever their area of interest or chosen practice method, become involved, in one way or another, with group leadership, coordination or facilitation. Whether it is leadership of a group therapy session, development of a community activist team, facilitation of a support group, direction of a poetry workshop, or management of a volunteer Board, social workers, everywhere, are called upon to utilize group work skills. This special volume, directed at group work with older persons, is thus a valuable publication for each one of us.

The very experience of reading the articles gives one the impression of becoming a group participant in a group populated by the authors. The reader learns specific knowledge and skills from peers, gains mutual support and validation for his/her own work, and is inspired and challenged. Welcome to the group.

M. Joanna Mellor, DSW

[Haworth co-indexing entry note]: "Foreword." Mellor, M. Joanna. Co-published simultaneously in *Journal of Gerontological Social Work* (The Haworth Social Work Practice Press, an imprint of The Haworth Press, Inc.) Vol. 44, No. 1/2, 2004, pp. xxv; and: *Group Work and Aging: Issues in Practice, Research, and Education* (ed: Robert Salmon, and Roberta Graziano) The Haworth Social Work Practice Press, an imprint of The Haworth Press, Inc., 2004, pp. xix. Single or multiple copies of this article are available for a fee from The Haworth Document Delivery Service [1-800-HAWORTH, 9:00 a.m. - 5:00 p.m. (EST). E-mail address: docdelivery@haworthpress.com].

xix

Introduction

This volume includes a series of articles that describe the complexity, diversity, and particular usefulness of social group work practice in the service of older adults-the aging and the aged. Some of the articles present examples of direct practice with specific groups of older clients. Others are concerned with the group work practice with caregivers or workers who devote their efforts to serving the elderly. The implicit foundation for all of the work is that social group work practice, throughout its history, structure, and approach, is a positive and optimistic way of working with people. "It is truly empowering and affirming of people's strengths . . . and in the contribution that each person can make to others' lives. In today's troubled world, effective group work is needed more than ever" (Kurland and Salmon, 1998, p. IX).

Social workers understand this, and they form and work with many kinds of groups including support groups, reminiscence and life review groups, socialization groups, cognitive behavioral groups, behavior modification groups, activity groups, therapy groups, task groups, supervisory and administrative groups, and psychoeducational groups, to name but a few. A common theme in all is the principle of mutual aid.

> Mutual aid is at the very heart of good group work practice. The expectation that members of a group will be able to help one another-in fact, they will be expected to do so-is a statement to each person in the group that she or he has strengths to offer to others . . . Mutual aid means that client strengths are called upon and empha-

[Haworth co-indexing entry note]: "Introduction." Salmon, Robert. Co-published simultaneously in *Journal of Gerontological Social Work* (The Haworth Social Work Practice Press, an imprint of The Haworth Press, Inc.) Vol. 44, No. 1/2, 2004, pp. 1-4; and: *Group Work and Aging: Issues in Practice, Research, and Education* (ed: Robert Salmon, and Roberta Graziano) The Haworth Social Work Practice Press, an imprint of The Haworth Press, Inc., 2004, pp. 1-4. Single or multiple copies of this article are available for a fee from The Haworth Document Delivery Service [1-800-HAWORTH, 9:00 a.m. - 5:00 p.m. (EST). E-mail address: docdelivery@haworthpress.com].

Digital Object Identifier: 10.1300/J083v44n01-01

sized, a feature that makes group work special and unique and wonderful. (Steinberg, 2004, p. XI)

A mutual aid approach to working with groups will be seen throughout the articles presented in this volume. It is inherent in the work.

Two articles buttress and reinforce all the other work that appears in this volume: the lead article by Ron Toseland and Victoria Rizzo, *"What's Different About Working with Older People in Groups,"* and the ending article, *"Remembering With and Without Awareness Through Poetry to Better Understand Aging and Disability,"* by Andrew Malekoff. Toseland and Rizzo, with great care and perceptiveness, discuss the adaptation of group work techniques and strategies for work with older adults and their unique developmental needs. They are educators and gerontologists. Toseland has published extensively in the group work literature. Their scholarly and comprehensive article reflects positively on the years of work, thinking and writing about group work with the aged.

Malekoff also has published extensively, and his subject matter is more likely to be about group work with adolescents. His poetry/article in this volume is personal and literary. It evokes his experience with his grandfathers and their disabilities. This shaped the interactions he has now with the aged and disabled. His poems about the death of his father in a hospital underscore the stress of making life-and-death decisions about another, and the need for the development of short-term, hospital-based mutual aid groups that could help in that painful process.

The category of support group provides a rubric for a broad range of groups with different purposes and populations. Four articles by Helene Ebenstein, Harriet Goodman, Ann Goelitz, and Smith, Toseland, Rizzo, and Zinoman describe diverse populations and varied client needs and issues. Their commonality is that the group members discussed in the articles all are caregivers of the aged. Goelitz, and Smith, Toseland, Rizzo, and Zinoman discuss telephone support groups. Caregivers, in particular, may find it difficult to come to meetings, and technology is used to conduct the work of the group. Even the Internet is being used at times for this purpose. These articles show the opportunities as well as the difficulties of offering effective help in a different way.

Over thirty years ago, Garfield and Irrizary (1971) wrote an article introducing the Record of Service (ROS) as a tool to be used by group workers for the examination of their practice. Hunter College School of Social Work group work faculty added to this tool over the years and use it now for the major assignments for advanced group work students. Kris Drumm led a support group with older women who are lesbians.

Using the ROS as a tool for accountability, practice examination, and skills enhancement, her article provides an exemplar for practicing group workers.

Substance abuse among older adults is discussed in the article by Guida, Unterbach, Tavolacci, and Provet. Their article includes the extensive research that led to the development of social group work as their primary treatment model.

Two articles concern mutual aid groups. Tim Kelly discusses his direct work with groups of older clients with a mental illness, and Sister Maria Theresa Amato wrote about her work with a group of home attendants employed to care for Alzheimer's patients by their families. Both groups, each in their own way, were vulnerable and unappreciated. The mutual aid approach was crucial for them in learning to deal with the issues and problems they faced.

The need for quality educational programs to produce the next generation of skilled group workers to work with the growing older population is imperative. Barbara Rinehart and Roberta Graziano discuss the effectiveness of using group supervision as the primary teaching tool with their experienced work-study MSW students who were providing services to the aged. Here, too, the mutual aid approach was essential to the learning process.

The use of program and activity always has been an intrinsic, albeit a sometimes controversial part of group work practice. Grace Coyle (1946) addressed this issue when she wrote:

> . . . Program and relationships are inextricably intertwined. Social group work method developed as we began to see that the understanding and the use of the human relations involved were as important as the understanding and use of various types of programs. (pp. 202-203)

Articles by Sarah Stevenson, Irene Chung, and Cusicanqui and Salmon discuss the use of program and activity as the means to achieve the goals of the group. The groups described were diverse. They include older homeless adults, Asian-American elderly immigrants, and an intergenerational group of older adults and children. Each article describes the group's sociocultural reality, and the practice problems involved in achieving the group's purpose. The achievement of their goals was inconceivable without the skillful and purposeful use of program activities.

This volume was also inconceivable without the willing participation of the authors of the fine articles in this collection. Roberta Graziano, a friend and colleague at Hunter, asked me to be the senior editor. Other Hunter colleagues, through their writing, contributed their wisdom and talent. Other contributors are group work graduates of Hunter, and several were my students over thirty years ago. Some are recent graduates, and one extraordinary participant (the youngest of the authors) will not graduate with her MSW degree until June 2005. Others are group workers who have contributed to the group work literature for many years. Several of the authors brought in their colleagues to work with them. Collectively they have created a very useful volume on group work and aging, which will have a positive effect on group work practice for years to come.

Robert Salmon, DSW

REFERENCES

Coyle, Grace (1946). "Social Group Work in Recreation." In *Proceedings of the National Conference of Social Work 1946* (pp. 202-203). New York: Columbia University Press.

Garfield, Goodwin, and Irrizary, Carol (1971). "The Record of Service: Describing Social Work Practice." In William Schwartz, and Serapio Zalba (Eds.), *The Practice of Group Work* (pp. 242- 261). New York: Columbia University Press.

Kurland, Roselle, and Salmon, Robert (1998). *Teaching a Methods Course in Social Work With Groups* (p. IX). Alexandria, VA: Council on Social Work Education.

Steinberg, Dominique M. (2004). *The Mutual-Aid Approach to Working with Groups: Helping People Help One Another*, 2nd ed. (p. XI). New York: The Haworth Press, Inc.

What's Different About Working with Older People in Groups?

Ronald W. Toseland, PhD

Victoria M. Rizzo, PhD

SUMMARY. Group work is a modality that is used extensively with older adults. This article reviews the literature about group work with older adults and describes adaptations that may be needed when working with groups of older people. These adaptations include considering the influence of age-related changes on members' abilities to participate in the group, how cohort effects change group dynamics, and understanding the impact of age-related developmental changes. The article then reviews themes that are frequent topics of interaction in groups of older persons. The article concludes with a review of indications and contraindications for group participation, how leadership may need to be adapted for work with certain groups of older persons, and how stages of group development are affected by the participation of older group members. *[Article copies available for a fee from The Haworth Document Delivery Service: 1-800-HAWORTH. E-mail address: <docdelivery@haworthpress.com> Website: <http://www.HaworthPress.com> © 2004 by The Haworth Press, Inc. All rights reserved.]*

KEYWORDS. Elderly, old age, age-related adaptations, adult development

---

[Haworth co-indexing entry note]: "What's Different About Working with Older People in Groups?" Toseland, Ronald W., and Victoria M. Rizzo. Co-published simultaneously in *Journal of Gerontological Social Work* (The Haworth Social Work Practice Press, an imprint of The Haworth Press, Inc.) Vol. 44, No. 1/2, 2004, pp. 5-23; and: *Group Work and Aging: Issues in Practice, Research, and Education* (ed: Robert Salmon, and Roberta Graziano) The Haworth Social Work Practice Press, an imprint of The Haworth Press, Inc., 2004, pp. 5-23. Single or multiple copies of this article are available for a fee from The Haworth Document Delivery Service [1-800-HAWORTH, 9:00 a.m. - 5:00 p.m. (EST). E-mail address: docdelivery@haworthpress. com].

http://www.haworthpress.com/web/JGSW
© 2004 by The Haworth Press, Inc. All rights reserved.
Digital Object Identifier: 10.1300/J083v44n01-02

Group work is a service modality that is used extensively with older adults in many different settings. A review of the literature from 1970 to 1996, however, revealed 451 articles, dissertations, and other publications about group work practice with older adults, a rate of only about nine published documents per year (Aday & Aday, 1997). Despite the modest amount of literature about group work with the elderly that appears each year, group workers facilitate many different types of treatment and task groups with elderly members in community and institutional settings.

A review of the literature since 1996 for this article revealed that group work with older adults can be focused on many different purposes. For example, treatment groups with elderly members can focus on activities (Pinquart, Wenzel, & Soerensen, 2000; Link, 1997; Yaretzky, Levinson, & Kimchi, 1996), education (Ersek, Turner, McCurry, Gibbons, & Kraybill; 2003; Brody, Williams, Thomas, Kaplan, Chu, & Brown, 1999; Ramos, Toseland, Smith, & McCallion, in press; Toseland, McCallion, Smith, Huck, Bourgeois, & Garstka, 2001), growth (Brown & Abby, 1999; Dube, Lapierre, Bouffard, & Labelle, 2000; Tennstedt, Lawrence, & Kasten, 2001), socialization (Ryan & Doubleday, 1995), support (Mueller & Barash-Kishon, 1998; Greenberg, Motenko, Roesch, & Embleton, 1999), recreation (Erwin, 1996), and therapy (Cooper & Doherty, 2000; Evans, Chisholm, & Walshe, 2001; Klausner, Snyder, & Cheavens, 2000; Molinari, 2002). Group work skills are also used when facilitating advocacy, service, and other types of task groups, such as committees, councils, and teams composed of older people.

Historically, most group work practice with older adults occurred in long-term social, recreational, and therapeutic groups in community and institutional settings (see, for example, Konopka, 1954; Kubie & Landau, 1953; Linden, 1953; Woods, 1953). More recently, however, there has been an increase in short-term psychoeducational groups (Toseland et al., 2001), reminiscence and life review groups (Link, 1997), self-help groups, and support groups (Mueller & Barash-Kishon, 1998; Greenberg et al., 1999) for older persons residing in community and institutionalized settings.

PREPARING FOR GROUP WORK WITH OLDER ADULTS

Most group workers lack personal experience with the developmental issues faced by older adults. When working with younger people, group work practitioners can draw from their own life experiences. But, when working with older persons, most group workers can only draw upon vicarious experiences with grandparents and other elders. Because of this lack of personal experience, it is often necessary for group work practitioners to sensitize themselves to the positive and negative aspects of aging, and to the developmental issues typically faced by older adults. To begin this process, it is helpful for workers to identify their own attitudes and feelings about aging. Like some other young and middle-aged persons who are not group work practitioners, group workers' images of aging may be distorted by negative stereotypes.

It is important for group workers to be aware of their own negative reactions to aging and how this might affect their group work practice. Grappling with age-related changes in physical appearance, reduced physical functioning, death, and so forth, can be challenging. Negative reactions and stereotypes can be exacerbated because group workers often work with older adults who are frail or disabled. Although groups of well older adults meet in senior citizens centers, senior housing and many other settings, in general, healthy elderly who are enjoying life are less likely to use group work services than are frail elderly living in community and institutional settings. Therefore, group workers should begin by examining their own stereotypes about aging, and their own reactions to growing older.

AGE-RELATED CHANGES

It is also important for group workers to understand the impact of age-related changes on the older people they are working with in groups. There is tremendous variability in age-related changes. Therefore, those who work with older persons in groups should be aware of the possibility of age-related changes, while at the same time carefully assessing individual variation. Physically, for example, the young-old who are in their 50s, 60s, and early 70s are often not appreciably affected by age-related physical changes. With increasing age (beyond the early 70s), however, the prevalence of chronic disabilities increases, and functional limitations become more common. With advancing age (85 years of age or older), there is a gradual slowing of reaction time and speed, and the acuity of the senses declines (Fozard & Gordon-Salant, 2001; Madden, 2001). Working memory also declines, but older people compensate with a storehouse of experience about how things work. Thus, these decrements in physical functioning often do not become severe enough to affect the day-to-day functioning of older adults until they reach advanced old age. Still, they can affect the pace of group meetings.

With respect to mental health, with the exception of dementia, older adults have lower rates of mental health problems than other age groups (Zarit & Zarit, 1998). Older adults may suffer, however, from a higher level of symptoms of depression than previously thought, and their rate of suicide is the highest of any age group (Department of Health and Human Services, 2003).

Emotionally, there is some evidence that older adults are more difficult to arouse, but that they also have more difficulty returning to a calm state once they are aroused (Woodruff, 1985). This suggests that older persons may avoid becoming emotionally aroused in groups, but when they become aroused, group workers may have to take more care to assure that they have returned to a calm state before leaving the group. There is also some evidence that older people's emotional lives are more complex than younger persons' with new experiences reminding older people of previous experiences that have a mix of positive and negative feelings attached to them (Schulz, 1982; Knight & McCallum, 1998). In this way, older people may be more able than younger persons to understand and appreciate the complexity of emotional feelings that can result from an emotionally charged event.

Socially, older adults lose roles as they age. For example, when older people retire they lose work-related roles. With advancing age, other losses occur, such as the death of longtime friends and spouses. At the same time, older adults often take on new roles, such as becoming grandparents, volunteering, or serving as caregivers. Social group work has an important role to play in helping older persons to cope with and adjust both to lost roles and to newly acquired roles.

COHORT EFFECTS ON GROUP DYNAMICS

Group workers should be aware of both the uniqueness of each older person they work with, as well as common developmental tasks and themes shared by older persons of different chronological ages. It is important for group workers to understand that with increasing age chronological age becomes less important because of the variable rates by which individuals age. Still, one way that chronological age plays a role in group dynamics is through cohort effects (Knight, 1996; Toseland, 1995). For example, a group of 80- to 90-year-olds share the experience of going through the economic depression of the 1930s. Because of this experience, these individuals may place more emphasis on thrift and economic security than those in their 60s. They also share other experiences, such as a world without television or computers and memories of World War II. In addition to shared memories and experiences, other cohort effects can affect group work. For example, older cohorts tend to be less well-educated than younger cohorts. Group workers, therefore, should check the reading level of handouts and should use less complex terminology when working with older cohorts than when working with younger cohorts. Similarly, mental health issues, counseling, etc., were less available and more stigmatized for older cohorts than for younger cohorts. Therefore, older cohorts are less likely to have a psychological worldview (Knight, 1996). Furthermore, they may be more hesitant to join group meetings and engage with others in groups because they do not want to be stigmatized or be seen as needing help. For example, one of the authors facilitated a cardiac education/support group in an inpatient rehabilitation setting. When she approached patients on the day of the group, many older patients would say, "I do not need to go to this group. I know some people need help, but I don't. I handle my problems on my own." However, when they agreed to go, participants were often surprised that they liked the group and learned how to better deal with stress using relaxation techniques and new coping strategies.

UNDERSTANDING DEVELOPMENTAL CHANGES

It is essential for group workers to understand developmental changes that occur with age. The literature clearly indicates that although personality continues to develop in old age, there is a great deal of continuity in personality traits over time (Ryff, Kwan, & Singer, 2001). This suggests that group leaders should make a point to find out about older adults' personality traits and build on them using a strengths-based, empowerment approach, rather than try to change traits established and set over a lifetime.

Despite a great deal of continuity, there are some developmental changes that occur as individuals grow old. For example, environmental mastery and autonomy become more important as people age, whereas purpose in life and personal growth tend to exhibit downward age trajectories (Ryff, Kwan, & Singer, 2001). Group work has an important role to play by helping older people to discuss and meet the challenges of maintaining environmental mastery and autonomy in the face of physical and psychological losses. Also, although ruminations about purpose in life and personal growth wane with age, the importance of group work for helping older people to view their lives as meaningful increases.

There are also differences in coping styles between young and old persons that have important implications for group work with older persons. Diehl, Coyle, and Labouvie-Vief (1996), for example, found that older people tended to use more varied coping strategies, to have greater impulse control, and to have a more positive appraisal of conflict situations. Younger people tended to use more aggressive and undifferentiated coping strategies, indicating lower levels of impulse control and less insight. There is also some evidence to suggest that older persons use more emotion-focused coping skills such as seeking social support, positive reappraisal and distancing, whereas younger people tend to use more problem-focused coping skills such as confrontation, information seeking, and problem solving (Folkman, Lazarus, Pimley, & Novacek, 1987). These findings suggest that there is likely to be less aggression and confrontation in groups of older persons than in groups of younger persons, and that the elderly may be less willing to accept suggestions for the use of active and assertive coping skills. Both of these observations are born out in our clinical experiences with groups of older persons.

More pronounced developmental changes occur in the very old. Tobin (1999) indicates that while the task of the earliest years is to become oneself, and the task of the adult years is to fulfill oneself, the task of the oldest years is to preserve the self. In order to maintain control and mastery, the oldest old tend to contract their personal environment and their interactions with others so as to maintain a sense of control and mastery albeit in a smaller physical and social arena. For example, an elderly woman in the Northeast may choose to store her car for the winter because she no longer feels she can go out alone in the ice and snow without falling or hurting herself. Another example is an individual's decision to no longer use the second floor of a home because she can no longer climb stairs easily and can better maintain her independence and her home by only using the first floor. There are also downward social comparisons, where older people compare themselves to those that are sicker or no longer alive. That is why older people will often say they are in good health or very good health even though they may have a number of chronic health problems. Another characteristic of the very old is their religiosity. Religion is a very important coping mechanism for many of the oldest old and they are more likely to discuss in groups the importance of religion in coping with stressful life events than are younger people.

Interiority is also more pronounced in the oldest old. The oldest old are concerned with accepting life and making sense of it as they have lived it. There is more blending of the past and the present than among younger persons. For example, an elderly group member who retired from a career as a carpenter some 30 years previously may still refer to himself as being a carpenter. Interiority also means that older people are often more concerned about bodily functions and physical changes than are younger persons. For example, in many of the groups conducted with individuals in hospital settings, the authors often found that frail elderly patients spent a great deal of time discussing changes in bowel movements in group sessions with each other and they placed great importance on this topic. Clinical experience suggests that the oldest old group members listen politely to others but are more concerned about what is going on inside them than what is going on with other members. In some groups, the interaction is akin to parallel play in children where children at certain ages play together but do not really interact. For example, when one group member describes a relationship issue she is having with her daughter rather than responding with problem-solving suggestions to the group member, older group members are more likely to describe relationship issues with their children without making a connection to the first group member's comments. Therefore, group work with older adults often requires leaders to be active in making connections between members and helping members to listen to and comment on each other's concerns. It also means giving older persons time to talk about their intrapersonal concerns.

Interiority can also take the form of reminiscence, placing previous life events in positive context, and even mythicizing the past and distorting past events to make them acceptable (Tobin, 1999). For example, their adult children may not view a group member as a very good parent. Nevertheless, the group member may view herself as a good parent, and parenting as one of the positive accomplishments of her life. Seeing herself as a mediocre or bad parent may simply not be an acceptable way of viewing her life. Through reminiscing, reflection, and group discussion, groups can help older people place their lives in a positive context. The implication also is that it may not be helpful for group workers or group members to challenge apparent distortions, or revisions of historical facts, but rather to help the very old consider and reflect on accomplishments, achievements, and how well they are coping in the face of losses.

THEMES IN GROUP MEETINGS

Although the experience of aging can be quite diverse, there are some themes that frequently come up when older adults meet together in groups. These themes include: (1) continuity with the past, (2) understanding the modern world, (3) independence, (4) physical and cognitive impairments, (5) loss of family members and friends, (6) spouses and other family of origin relationships, (7) children and grandchildren, (8) resources, (9) environmental vulnerability and adjustment, (10) religious conviction and ethnic pride, and (11) leisure pursuits (Toseland, 1995).

The theme, continuity with the past, means that many older adults enjoy talking about their past accomplishments and what life has been like for them. Recalling, reliving, and reminiscing about past experiences enables older persons to share their experience and wisdom with others. Many selectively remember those events that were particularly pleasurable and that give their life meaning (Tobin, 1999). Groups can serve as a useful forum for reminiscence and for selectively remembering and reframing past events.

The theme, understanding the modern world, means that older people often use groups to help themselves understand and adapt to the world, which has changed so dramatically from when they were young. Groups help by enabling older persons to interact with peers who share similar historical experiences, and who affirm the importance of these experiences.

The themes, independence, physical and cognitive impairments, and loss of family members and friends, are interrelated. Older persons worry about becoming dependent, and physical and cognitive impairments are threats to their independence. Similarly, losses of family members and friends are also viewed as threats to independence. Loss is a theme that frequently comes up when older people meet in groups (Burnside & Schmidt, 1994). Therefore, group work practitioners who work with older people should be familiar with grieving processes and healthy adjustments to loss.

Family relationships, including relationships with children and grandchildren, take on added importance for older persons because of the loss of other social roles and relationships, changes in marital relationships brought about by retirement, and increased dependence on family for help with chronic health problems. Groups can be helpful by encouraging members to reflect on changing family relationships. They can also help older adults consider what can be realistically expected from spouses and other family members in the present and the future. Groups can help older adults to explore how relationships can be improved or strengthened, and when it may be helpful to supplement or extend informal care with formal care by professional caregivers.

Living on fixed incomes makes many older persons keenly aware of the resources they have at their disposal. Inflation and health problems that have a negative impact on budgets are frequent topics of conversation when older people meet together in groups. Groups can help by making older people aware of programs such as Supplemental Security Income, food stamps, meals on wheels, home heating assistance, reverse home loans, home repair, and other aid programs. Group members and the leader also can share information about other programs that may indirectly affect older adult resources. These programs include case management, congregate meals, day care, health screening programs, home care, senior center, senior transportation, and other government, voluntary, and for-profit programs designed to help older people to maintain their independence for as long as possible.

As people age they become more vulnerable to perceived changes in their environment. In groups, older people discuss changes in their community and their individual life circumstances that threaten their well-being. Issues such as losing one's ability to drive and difficulties in maintaining one's residence, are frequently discussed when groups of seniors meet. Support groups can provide an empathic environment where older adults can discuss their feelings of vulnerability and gain support from one another. Groups can also help older persons to sustain feelings of mastery and control by providing them with a social support network, and a place where mutual aid can be exchanged.

Religious conviction and ethnic pride lend resiliency to elderly group members who may be burdened by disabilities and losses. Groups provide an opportunity for members to discuss their religious conviction, and their pride in their ethnic backgrounds and traditions. Clinical experience from listening to hundreds of audiotapes of group sessions resulting from research on group work with older people, leads us to conclude that, too often, group workers do not pay enough attention to the role of religion, spirituality, and ethnic pride in the lives of older group members.

Leisure pursuits are also an important theme in groups of older persons. Educational and recreational groups are common in senior centers and other community agencies. Groups enable members to spend time productively, following up on interests and hobbies that they may not have been able to pursue earlier in life, and to engage in new social roles.

INDICATIONS AND CONTRAINDICATIONS
FOR GROUP PARTICIPATION

There are many benefits for older persons who participate in groups. These include: (1) belonging and affiliation, (2) consensual validation and affirmation of one's experiences, (3) ventilation, (4) satisfying and meaningful roles, (5) interpersonal learning, (6) information, (7) problem solving, and (8) support. Groups are particularly well-suited for older persons who are socially isolated and for those who need help in identifying and participating in new social roles. Groups enable older people to interact with each other and to take on new roles. Groups are also particularly helpful for those who have interpersonal problems. Peer feedback, reality testing, role models, and suggestions for how to behave can all be helpful for older people with interpersonal problems.

There are at least three barriers to group participation among older adults including: (1) practical barriers, (2) certain therapeutic needs, and (3) disabilities. Practical barriers are probably the single most important reason why more group work is not done with older persons. With increasing age, it is harder for older people to get to face-to-face groups. They may no longer drive, they may not feel they have the physical stamina to attend group meetings, or they may feel that they are needed at home to do informal caregiving for a spouse. In recent years, there has been a growing interest in teleconferencing, and web-based technologies to overcome these practical barriers (Rizzo & Toseland, 2003; Galinsky, Schopler, & Abell, 1997; Schopler, Abell, & Galinsky, 1998; Kaslyn, 1999; Smokowski, Galinsky, & Harlow, 2001; and Stein, Rothman, & Nakanishi, 1993).

Certain therapeutic needs may also contraindicate or place barriers on the receipt of group work services. For example, older persons who are in crisis may be served more effectively in individual therapy, at least until they can get the concentrated help they need to stabilize a crisis. Older people who have highly personal or idiosyncratic problems may be better off in individual therapy.

Although cognitively and physically impaired older persons can be successfully served by participating in social work groups, disabilities can present problems and challenges for group workers. For example, in most cases, cognitively intact and cognitively impaired older adults should not be placed in the same group. Separate groups often need to be developed to meet disparate needs of these two populations. Similarly, although people with visual and hearing impairments can be successfully served in groups (see, for example, Horowitz, Leonard, &

Reinhardt, 2000), these impairments can be barriers to group participation.

LEADERSHIP OF OLDER ADULT GROUPS

Because of the tremendous variability of the aging population, one should be very cautious about making generalizations about what is different about leading groups of older persons. One important consideration, however, concerns the pace of group meetings, and the speed and timing of interventions. In general, as age increases, and cognitive and physical disabilities increase, the pace of group meetings should be slowed. A greater emphasis should be placed on using wisdom and experience rather than learning new information. However, when new information is needed or desired, slowed interaction patterns, repetition and simplification, the use of many senses to convey information, and linking with past experiences about learning new knowledge, can be helpful strategies depending on the age and cognitive and physical disability of those involved in the group. Toseland and McCallion (1998), for example, have developed a number of communication strategies for maintaining interaction with cognitively impaired persons, including those who display agitated behavior and other challenging behaviors.

Another important consideration is the content of group meetings. With increasing age, group leaders may want to encourage and support older adults to use autobiography, Delese, 1991; reminiscence, and other life review strategies (see, for example, Birren & Deutchman, 1991; Birren, Kenyon, Ruth, Schroots, & Svensson, 1996; Gibson, 2004; Kenyons, Clark, & deVries, 2001; Link, 1997; Webster & Haight, 2002) so that they can put their life in perspective. Remotivation and reality orientation program activities are other commonly-used methods that affect the content of group meetings (Link, 1997). More attention should also be paid to issues focused on continuity between the past and the present, and to cohort similarities and differences among members. Knight and colleagues (Knight, 1996; Knight & McCallum, 1998) also point out that older persons face specific challenges such as chronic illness and disability, grieving, and caregiving that are less common among younger persons.

A third consideration is the extent to which the social group worker shares leadership, and empowers older adults to achieve their own goals. While empowerment is important for working with groups of all ages, unlike when working with young persons, older people bring a wealth of experience and wisdom to groups that have been garnered over a lifetime of living. For the well elderly, this means that social group workers should bring out the experience and wisdom of group members and also their leadership capabilities. For very old or frail elderly, group leaders may have to be very active in order to make connections between members. Still, empowerment means that it is important to help these older people to utilize and shore-up longstanding coping skills to address current life situations. In general, empowerment strategies encourage older adults to bring previous life experiences to groups, to assert informal leadership, and to take control over what they want to get out of the group experience.

A fourth consideration is how group workers engage older persons in behavior change and coping. Older people draw on a wealth of experience in dealing with problems and issues in their lives. They have developed ways of coping and ways of changing to accommodate to the many different circumstances they have found themselves to be in over the years. At the same time, previously mentioned research indicates that older persons tend to be less aggressive and less likely to confront problems directly. They are also more likely to use more passive coping skills than younger persons. Therefore, adaptations may be needed in cognitive behavioral and other psychoeducational approaches that encourage older people to use new and more active coping skills (see, for example, Brok, 1997). New coping skills approaches should be placed within the context of older group members' previous attempts to resolve problems and issues they have faced in the past. Older people may need more time to explain how they have coped in the past, and to reflect on the wisdom of using new coping skills. New coping skills may be modified to fit the older person's experience in previous situations.

A fifth leadership consideration is the social context in which older people live and groups take place. Knight and McCallum (1998) point out that those who work with older adults should be familiar with the aging service network in the areas where older persons live. Group workers also need to know about the way that particular environments, such as senior housing or nursing homes, can affect elderly group members. For example, in senior housing it is not uncommon for residents to refuse to participate in a group if they find that another resident, who they dislike, is planning to participate. Similarly, group workers in nursing homes should be aware of how high levels of cognitive impairment and loss of autonomy affect residents.

STAGES OF GROUP DEVELOPMENT

Like groups of younger persons, groups of older persons go through distinct stages of development. According to Toseland and Rivas (in press) there are four distinct stages of group development: (1) planning, (2) beginning, (3) middle, and (4) ending. In this article, we will not cover all of these phases in depth but will instead highlight key elements in each stage that set group work with older adults apart from group work with younger persons.

One of the aspects of the planning stage of group work with older persons that differs from work with younger persons is preparing the group's environment and making special arrangements. Because older persons may have chronic health problems or functional disabilities, it is especially important to ensure that groups are held in comfortable locations with handicap access. Group workers should consider such factors as whether the meeting room is accessible to wheelchairs, whether there are stairs to climb, and whether aids to walking, such as handrails, will be needed. Because older people may have trouble getting in and out of low chairs, it is preferable to have high back armchairs of standard height. Bathroom facilities that are close to the group meeting room and accessible are also of particular importance when conducting groups with elderly individuals. For example, bathrooms should have grab bars, raised toilet seats, and wide doorways for wheelchairs. Noise and other distractions are particularly problematic for older persons who may have some hearing loss. Therefore, it is important to keep background noise to a minimum and to have good lighting. It is also often helpful to have a blackboard, an easel, and other learning aides that can convey ideas visually as well as verbally. Special arrangements, such as transportation, may also have to be planned in preparation for group work with older persons.

Another aspect of the planning stage that differs when working with older persons is the source of referrals and community resources and services that may be needed by older group members. With respect to recruiting members for a group, there are often small circulation, specialized newspapers and newsletters that focus on the elderly. Older persons are also more likely to enroll in a group if they are assured about the quality of the proposed group by persons within the aging network, such as senior housing managers, or senior center staff. To ensure that older people will get the services and resources they need, group workers who work with older adults should familiarize themselves with the aging services network in their community, including eligibility requirements for service delivery, and knowledge about how to make referrals.

During the beginning phase of group work, those who work with older adults may find that older persons tend to pay more attention, and to show greater respect for the group worker's credentials than do younger persons. It is unclear if this is a cohort effect where older cohorts tend to have greater respect for advanced degrees and credentials than do younger persons, or whether this is the result of neglected older adults wanting to be appreciated and valued by the leader for what they have accomplished in their lives. Notwithstanding the fact that older persons tend to show more respect and deference to the group leader than do younger persons, clinical experience suggests that some older persons treat group workers in a maternalistic or paternalistic fashion. For example, Poggi and Berland (1985) reported feeling angry, emasculated and unskilled when they were referred to by older group members as "dear," "honey," or as "sweet young boy or girl." When these expressions arise in groups, it may be helpful for the group worker to view them as endearments that attempt to personalize and make less formal members' relationships with the group worker, rather than as attempts to diminish the workers' authority or expertise (Toseland, 1995).

In groups of older adults it is particularly helpful to encourage older persons to share their wisdom and experience. Because some older persons share their wisdom and experience without connecting their thoughts to what others have been expressing, group workers should take an active stance, encouraging members to connect with each other by listening to and reacting to what others are expressing. Thus, although there tends to be less acting out and less testing of boundaries than when working with groups of younger persons, the worker still needs to take an active stance by connecting members and helping members to express themselves.

With respect to leadership during the beginning phase, there is a limited amount of evidence that indicates that older adults may benefit more than younger persons from an accepting, encouraging, supportive, and non-confrontational leadership approach where there is an emphasis on clarification and amplification of feelings (Lakin, Oppenheimer, & Bremer, 1982; Lazarus et al., 1984). These findings support studies mentioned previously indicating that older adults tend to rely more on emotion-focused coping skills than do younger persons, and that older persons resist being emotionally aroused in groups and find it harder to return to a calm state once they are aroused.

Adaptations of the middle phase of group work depend very much on the capacities and capabilities of the older persons who are involved in a particular group, as well as the purpose of the group meeting. When working with groups of the young old, most group workers will find that they have to make few adaptations. However, as group members become older and frailer, adaptations often become more pronounced. For example, the pace of meetings may be slowed, and the worker may have to be more active in leading the group and making connections between members. Also, there may be more emphasis on reminiscence and life review and more use of specialized interventions such as reality orientation or remotivation therapy for the severely impaired (Folsom, 1968; Weiner, Brok, & Snadowsky, 1987).

There is very little information in the group work literature about the ending stage of group work with older adults. Clinical experience suggests that older adults show less emotion, and engage in less acting out behavior during the ending phase of group work than do younger persons. At the same time, the group worker should be aware that older people, particularly the very old, often experience more losses than do younger persons. It is not uncommon to hear older persons, who are in their late 80s and 90s, talking about the fact that most of their lifelong friends and companions have died. Despite less outward emotion, the termination, or end, of a group may be experienced by some older persons as another loss. Therefore, it can be helpful to end groups gradually, expanding the time between meetings but continuing follow-up meetings for some time. It can also be helpful to encourage members to get together between meetings. For example, in one group program for spouse caregivers of frail older persons, members were encouraged to exchange telephone numbers in early group sessions, and to call fellow members between meetings to share information, encouragement, and support (Toseland et al., 2001). It was found that an open invitation to telephone other members between meetings was not always successful. Members were reluctant to "call and bother other members with their problems." Telephone interaction between meetings was much more successful when group members were encouraged to plan during meetings who they were going to call, and what time and day the call would be made. Some groups from this and other group work programs for the elderly decided to continue to meet without the worker, usually in informal settings such as a group members' home, or at a local restaurant. Although these meetings were less frequent than the formal group meetings led by the worker, they served to extend members' social networks, and to prevent members from experiencing the formal ending of meetings as another "loss."

CONCLUSION

Group work with older persons is both as challenging and rewarding as group work with younger persons. Adaptation of group work techniques and strategies for work with older adults should first and foremost consider the unique developmental needs of older adults. Although there is tremendous variability among older adults that always should be taken into consideration, this article has described some themes that are commonly found in groups of older persons, and some leadership adaptations that may be needed when working with certain groups of older persons. These themes and adaptations are often less pronounced when working with young older persons than when working with the very old, and those in poor health with disabilities and functional limitations.

REFERENCES

Aday, R. H., & Aday, K. L. (1997). Group work with the elderly: An annotated bibliography. Westport, CT: Greenwood.

Birren, J., & Deutchman, D. (1991). Guiding autobiography groups for older adults: Exploring the fabric of everyday life. Baltimore, MD: Johns Hopkins.

Birren, J. E., Kenyon, G. M., Ruth, J. E., Schroots, J. J. F., & Svensson, T. (Eds.) (1996). *Aging and biography: Explorations in adult development.* New York: Springer.

Brody, B. L., Williams, R. A., Thomas, R. G., Kaplan, R. M., Chu, R. M., & Brown, S. I. (1999). Age related macular degeneration: A randomized clinical trial of a self-management intervention. *Annals of Behavioral Medicine, 21* (4), 322-329.

Brok, A. J. (1997). A modified cognitive-behavioral approach to group therapy with the elderly. *Group, 21* (2), 115-134.

Brown, W., & Abby, V. (1999). *Still kicking: Restorative groups for frail older adults.* Baltimore, MD: Health Professions Press.

Burnside, I., & Schmidt, M. G. (1994). *Working with older adults: Group process and techniques* (3rd edition). Boston, MA: Jones and Bartlett.

Cooper, C., & Doherty, J. (2000). Group work for older people with mental health problems. *Nursing Times, 96* (43), 42.

Department of Health and Human Services (2003). National Strategy for Suicide Prevention. Retrieved December 4, 2003, http://www.mentalhealth.org/suicideprevention/elderly.asp.

Diehl, M., Coyle, N., & Labouvie-Vief, G. (1996). Age and sex differences in strategies of coping and defense across the life span. *Psychology and Aging, 11,* 127-139.

Dube, M., Lapierre, S., Bouffard, L., & Labelle, R. (2000). Psychological well-being through the management of personal goals: A group intervention for retirees. *Revue-Quebecoise de Psychologie, 21* (2), 255-280.

Ersek, M., Turner, J. A., McCurry, S. M., Gibbons, L., & Kraybill, B. M. (2003). Efficacy of a self-management group intervention for elderly persons with chronic pain. *Clinical Journal of Pain, 19* (3), 156-167.

Erwin, K. T. (1996). *Group techniques for aging adults: Putting geriatric skills enhancement into practice.* Washington: Taylor and Francis.

Evans, S., Chisholm, P., & Walshe, J. (2001). A dynamic psychotherapy group for the elderly. *Group Analysis, 34* (2), 287-298.

Folkman, S., Lazarus, R., Pimley, S., & Novacek, J. (1987). Age differences in stress and coping processes. *Psychology and Aging, 2* (2), 171-184.

Folsom, J. C. (1968). Reality orientation for the elderly mental patient. *Journal of Geriatric Psychology, 1*, 291-307.

Fozard, J. L., & Gordon-Salant, S. (2001). Changes in vision and hearing with aging. In J. E. Birren & K. W. Schaie (Eds.), *Handbook of the psychology of aging* (5th edition, pp. 241-266). San Diego, CA: Academic Press.

Galinsky, M., Schopler, J., & Abell, M. (1997). Connecting group members through telephone and computer groups. *Health & Social Work, 22* (3), 181-188.

Gibson, F. (2004). *The past in the present: Using reminiscence.* Health Professions Press.

Greenberg, S., Motenko, A. K., Roesch, C., & Embleton, N. (1999). Friendship across the life cycle: A support group for older women. *Journal of Gerontological Social Work, 32* (4), 7-23.

Horowitz, A., Leonard, R., & Reinhardt, J. P. (2000). Measuring psychosocial and functional outcomes of a group model of vision rehabilitation services for older adults. *Journal of Visual Impairment and Blindness, 94* (5), 328-337.

Kaslyn, M. (1999). Telephone group work: Challenges for practice. *Social Work with Groups, 22*, 63-77.

Kenyon, G. M., Clark, P. G., & DeVries, B. (Eds.) (2001). *Narrative gerontology: Theory, research, and practice.* New York: Springer.

Klausner, E. J., Snyder, C. R., & Cheavens, J. (2000). A hope-based group treatment for depressed older adult outpatients. In G. M. Williamson & D. R. Shaffer (Eds.), *Physical illness and depression in older adults: A handbook of theory, research, and practice.* Dordrecht, The Netherlands: Kluwer Academic Publishers.

Knight, B. G. (1996). Psychotherapy with older adults (2nd edition). Thousand Oaks, CA: Sage.

Knight, B. G., & McCallum, T. J. (1998). Adapting psychotherapeutic practice to older clients: Implications of the contextual, cohort-based, maturity-specific challenge model. *Professional Psychology: Research and Practice, 29* (1), 15-22.

Konopka, G. (1954). Social group work in institutions for the aged. In G. Konopka (Ed.), *Group work in the institution: A modern challenge* (pp. 276-285). New York: Whiteside and Morrow.

Kubie, S., & Landau, G. (1953). *Group work with the aged.* New York: International Universities Press.

Lakin, M., Oppenheimer, B., & Bremer, J. (1982). A note on old and young in helping groups. *Psychotherapy: Theory, Research and Practice, 19*, 444-452.

Lazarus, L., Groves, L., Newton, N., Gutmann, D., Piceckyj, H., Frankel, R., Grunes, J., & Havasy-Galloway, S. (1984). Brief psychotherapy with the elderly: A review and preliminary study of process and outcome. In L. Lazarus (Ed.), *Clinical approaches to psychotherapy with the elderly* (pp. 15-35). Washington, DC: American Psychiatric Press.

Linden, M. (1953). Group psychotherapy with institutionalized senile women: Study in gerontological human relations. *International Journal of Group Psychotherapy, 3*, 150-170.

Link, A. L. (1997). *Group work with elders: 50 therapeutic exercises for reminiscence, validation, and remotivation.* Sarasota, FL: Professional Resource Press.

Madden, D. J. (2001). Speed and timing of behavioral processes. In J. E. Birren & K. W. Schaie (Eds.), *Handbook of the psychology of aging* (5th ed., pp. 288-312). San Diego: Academic Press.

Molinari, V. (2002). Group therapy in long term care sites. *Clinical Gerontologist, 25* (1/2), 13-24.

Mueller, U., & Barash-Kishon, R. (1998). Psychodynamic-supportive group therapy model for elderly Holocaust survivors. *International Journal of Group Psychotherapy, 48* (4), 461-475.

Pinquart, M., Wenzel, S., & Soerensen, S. (2000). Changes in attitude among children and elderly adults in intergenerational group work. *Educational Gerontology, 26* (6), 523-540.

Poggi, R., & Berland, D. (1985). The therapist's reactions to the elderly. *The Gerontologist, 25* (5), 508-513.

Ramos, B., Toseland, R., Smith, T., & McCallion, P. (In press). Latino family caregivers of the elderly: A health education program. *Social Work.*

Rizzo, V., & Toseland, R. (2003). *Leading telephone caregiver support groups: A manual for a model psychoeducational program.* Albany, NY: Institute of Gerontology, University at Albany, State University of New York.

Ryan, D., & Doubleday, E. (1995). Group work: A lifeline for isolated elderly. *Social Work with Groups, 18* (2-3), 65-78.

Ryff, C. D., Kwan, C. M. L., & Singer, B. H. (2001). Personality and aging: Flourishing agendas and future challenges. In J. E. Birren, & K. W. Schaie (Eds.), *Handbook of the psychology of aging* (5th edition, pp. 477-499). San Diego: Academic Press.

Schopler, J., Abell, M., & Galinsky, M. (1998). Technology-based groups: A review and conceptual framework for practice. *Social Work, 43* (3), 254-267.

Schulz, R. (1982). Emotionality and aging: A theoretical and empirical analysis. *Journal of Gerontology, 37*, 42-51.

Smokowski, P. R., Galinsky, M., & Harlow, C. K. (2001). Using technologies in group work, part II: Technology based groups. *Groupwork, 13* (1), 98-115.

Tennstedt, S. L., Lawrence, R. H., & Kasten, L. (2001). An intervention to reduce fear of falling and enhance activity: Who is most likely to benefit? *Educational Gerontology, 27* (3-4), 227-240.

Tobin, S. S. (1999). *Preservation of the self in the oldest years with implications for practice.* New York: Springer Publishing Company.

Toseland, R.W. (1995). *Group work with the elderly and family caregivers.* New York: Springer Publishing.

Toseland, R., & McCallion, P. (1998). *Maintaining communication with persons with dementia.* New York: Springer (Also includes workbook and 40-minute videotape).

Toseland, R., & Rivas, R. (in press). *An introduction to group work practice* (5th ed.). Boston: Allyn and Bacon.

Toseland, R., McCallion, P., Smith, T., Huck, S., Bourgeois, P., & Garstka, T. (2001). Health education groups for caregivers in an HMO. *Journal of Clinical Psychology, 57* (4), 551-570.

Webster, J., & Haight, B. K. (Eds.) (2002). *Critical advances in reminiscence work: From theory to application.* New York: Springer.

Weiner, M. B., Brok, A. J., & Snadowsky, A. M. (1987). *Working with the aged: Practical approaches in the institution and community* (2nd edition). Norwalk, CT: Appleton Century Crofts.

Woodruff, D. S. (1985). Arousal, sleep, and aging. In J. E. Birren & K. W. Schaie (Eds.), *Handbook of the psychology of aging* (2nd edition, pp. 261-295).

Woods, J. (1953). *Helping older people enjoy life.* New York: Harper.

Yaretzky, A., Levinson, M., & Kimchi, O. L. (1996). Clay as a therapeutic tool in group processing with the elderly. *American Journal of Art Therapy, 34* (3), 75-82.

Zarit, S. H., & Zarit, J. M. (1998). *Mental disorders in older adults: Fundamentals of assessment and treatment.* New York: The Guilford Press.

An Examination of Group Work
with Old Lesbians
Struggling with a Lack of Intimacy
by Using a Record of Service

Kris Drumm, MSW

SUMMARY. This article portrays the struggles old lesbians face in creating intimate friendships by using a Record of Service (ROS) of a support group. Using the ROS as an analytical tool, this paper demonstrates the efficacy of group work with this client population. The article also offers an explanation of the uses and mechanisms of the Record of Service and proffers it as a tool for accountability, practice examination, and skills improvement. Two sessions of a weekly support group for lesbians over sixty-years-old, conducted at SAGE (Senior Action in a Gay Environment), are excerpted to give the reader a personal view of this unique population as well as the practice of group work and the use of ROS. In the concluding analysis, the author critiques her interventions as well as the progress of the group. *[Article copies available for a fee from The Haworth Document Delivery Service: 1-800-HAWORTH. E-mail address: <docdelivery@haworthpress.com> Website: <http://www.HaworthPress.com> © 2004 by The Haworth Press, Inc. All rights reserved.]*

[Haworth co-indexing entry note]: "An Examination of Group Work with Old Lesbians Struggling with a Lack of Intimacy by Using a Record of Service." Drumm, Kris. Co-published simultaneously in *Journal of Gerontological Social Work* (The Haworth Social Work Practice Press, an imprint of The Haworth Press, Inc.) Vol. 44, No. 1/2, 2004, pp. 25-52; and: *Group Work and Aging: Issues in Practice, Research, and Education* (ed: Robert Salmon, and Roberta Graziano) The Haworth Social Work Practice Press, an imprint of The Haworth Press, Inc., 2004, pp. 25-52. Single or multiple copies of this article are available for a fee from The Haworth Document Delivery Service [1-800-HAWORTH, 9:00 a.m. - 5:00 p.m. (EST). E-mail address: docdelivery@haworthpress.com].

KEYWORDS. Record of Service (ROS), old, lesbians, senior, group work, intimacy

INTRODUCTION

This article brings the voices of old lesbians to the reader in the form of a Record of Service (ROS). It provides a unique glimpse of a weekly support group for lesbians over sixty-years-old at SAGE (Senior Action in a Gay Environment), which is located in New York City. Using the ROS as a lens, this paper will examine the efficacy of group work with this client population. The article also offers a description of what a Record of Service is and explains its uses and mechanisms, and proffers it as a tool for accountability, practice examination, and skills improvement.

BACKGROUND

Old lesbian activists at SAGE (Senior Action in a Gay Environment) have instructed me to use the word "old" instead of "senior" or other euphemisms because they are reclaiming "old" as a positive term rather than a pejorative one. In an ageist and heterosexist culture, they are often faced with pejorative images of themselves.

According to a report, issued by the NGLTF Policy Institute, on lesbian, gay, bisexual, and transgendered (LGBT) aging, nursing homes in this country document widespread homophobia among those providing care. As a result old LGBT people don't access health care, affordable housing, and other social services (Cahill, South, & Spade, 2000). Berkman and Zinberg (1997) discuss heterosexism and homophobia as the personal bias that social workers name as the hardest to overcome in providing services. A need for education and sensitivity about the lives of LGBT people is evident.

While many strides are being taken in the liberation and civil rights of LGBT people, LGBT people still face rampant homophobia and heterosexism. This oppression is manifested in verbal and physical assault on the street, discrimination in employment and housing, loss of custody and visitation rights of their children, and abandonment by family and friends (Greene, 1994). It is only within the last decade that LGBT people are beginning to see themselves more positively in media images, and those are young, white, and middle-class. It was not until this past year that the Supreme Court decriminalized same sex relationships.

Old LGBT people grew up in a society where laws disempowered, marginalized, criminalized, and pathologized them. Medical and mental health institutions often served as oppressive enforcers of these laws. In 1973 and 1988 respectively, the American Psychiatric Association removed the diagnosis of "homosexuality" and "ego dystonic homosexuality" from the DSMIV.

Cahill, South, and Spade (2000) estimate that there are anywhere from one to three million LGBT seniors living in the United States. However, since this population is made hidden and invisible by heterosexism and homophobia, it becomes difficult to validate these figures. Along with their more personal issues, the women's voices heard in the record of service to follow reflect the impact of being old and "queer."

THE RECORD OF SERVICE

Garfield and Irizarry (1971) designed the Record of Service (ROS) to be used as a tool for examination of social group work practice. The need for accountability and a systematic method of quality control were factors motivating its development. Since its inception, the formulation of the ROS has been honed by group social workers and teachers of group work to include a particular examination of the interventions that are used by practitioners in satisfying the purpose of the group (Getzel, Kurland, & Salmon, 1987). The skills described and discussed by Middleman and Wood (1990) are used for this purpose. Supervision, self-assessment, recordkeeping of group and individual progress, and quality control are uses for the ROS (Garfield & Irizarry, 1971; Getzel, Kurland, & Salmon, 1987).

Today, managed care has forced social workers to a new level of accountability and is pressuring them to employ "evidence-based practice" (Pollio, 2002, p. 59). Records of Service provide a performance measurement of the progress of the group, the individuals, and the worker.

Group work is complex with a myriad of considerations. Social group workers simultaneously must attend to four entities: the group, the individual, the relationship to each, and their relationship to worker. Each group is a unique organism, with its own life cycle of stages and role assumptions (Northen & Kurland, 2001; Shulman, 1999). The stage that a group is in will determine the amount of control the practitioner exercises as well as her expectations of work from the group (Shulman, 1999).

These complex dynamics are created within the context of the agency and the milieu of culture, positionality, and individual developmental stages. An understanding of power relationships, commonalities, and differences is gained in applying critical consciousness to these contextual elements (Reed, Newman, Suarez, & Lewis, 1997). Positionality locates people within the societal hierarchy of privilege and power, which determines to what degree participants experience external and internalized oppression (Reed et al., 1997). In examining our practice, locating our own positionality as well as our client's expands our awareness about the biases and assumptions, or the standpoints our relative experiences have given us.

Basic Procedure for Records of Service

In creating a social group work ROS, the worker begins by specifying the group type and purpose, the number of participants and the gender and age range of the group (Garfield & Irizarry, 1971; Getzel, Kurland & Salmon, 1987). The group task is then identified. Four major group tasks categorize the collective work of a social work group (Garfield & Irizarry, 1971; Getzel, Kurland, & Salmon, 1987). They are as follows: *Group formation*–which includes beginning stage problems such as establishing purpose; *group structure*–deals with more of the middle stage group issues, such as dealing with conflict and problem-solving processes; *relation to environment*–problems that concern the group's interaction with outside organizations or the sponsoring agency; and the fourth category, *group needs satisfaction*–helping the group deal with common identified themes. This specificity in delineating and defining the problem enables the practitioner to clearly conceptualize the issue they wish to focus on in the ROS.

After the group type, purpose, demographics, and group problem task are noted, the practitioner relates how the problem came to their attention, and how the group members are experiencing it. Following the problem identification is a summary of work wherein the practitioner excerpts as accurately as possible, interactions that portray the problem and the workers' response. Interactions that are the most challenging for the worker are purposefully detailed. The temptation to put only one's shining moments on paper must be resisted for the ROS to be fully effective. Reid (1997) suggests that in group work, one must display qualities including courage, honesty, self-knowledge, and humility (pp. 98-99). These attributes are necessary in creating an objective Record of Service.

The summary of work looks at how the problem is dealt with in a single session or many sessions. Ideally, interactions to be focused on have been documented immediately following each session while the content is fresh in the worker's mind. In creating a ROS, workers underline each intervention they make to differentiate it from their description which identifies the technique and skill used by the worker in that moment (Getzel, Kurland, & Salmon, 1987). The identification of skills is placed in italics above the underlined passages.

By identifying the skills that are employed in each intervention, social group workers are forced to think analytically about their responses and their lack of responses (Getzel, Kurland, & Salmon, 1987). The workers are then able to objectively evaluate their patterns, strengths and weaknesses in practice as well as their many clients' progress and patterns. The next step taken in the ROS is comprehensively identifying the next steps to be taken (Garfield & Irizarry, 1971; Getzel, Kurland, & Salmon, 1987). In addition to determining next steps, the ROS requires conceptualizing the theory behind the practitioner's use of skills.

The following ROS offers a frozen tableau that allows the observer to study how the SAGE Women's Support Group is grappling with the issue of emotional closeness as well as the effectiveness of my responses as the worker.

RECORD OF SERVICE

Group Type and Purpose. Old Lesbian's Support Group. An open, ongoing mutual-aid group whose purpose is to provide a place where lesbians over sixty can talk personally about issues affecting their lives and get support from each other.

Demographics. Age range is sixty- to eighty-years-old. Primarily white, mostly middle-class, lesbians. Numbers of women attending the group are usually between nine and twelve.

Group Task. Group needs satisfaction.

Problem. To help members identify and overcome obstacles that prevent them from being emotionally close with others.

Loneliness and Longing: How the Problem Came to My Attention

In the course of my four years tenure at SAGE, Senior Action in a Gay Environment, the issue of loneliness and desire for more "meaningful" friendships was a theme often mentioned by individual and group clients. Many of their friends have died or moved away. One woman spoke to the group about losing her partner of thirty-two years, and the strangeness she felt in reaching out to people now. This is not uncommon. Ruth, who is in her eighties, told the group she lost her partner of forty years and she "forgot how to make friends." Other members of the group echoed similar feelings. Some lesbians, gay men, bi-sexual and transgender SAGE members report not "coming out" as LGBT people until their later years, and losing family and community support upon doing so. For others, retirement created time they never had before, time often punctuated by a sense of loneliness and isolation. The desire for more meaningful and intimate friendships was identified by all members of the women's support group as a crucial one that they wanted to explore.

Summary of Work

This record of service documents excerpts from two sessions of the group. At this time, the group has met weekly for four months and a core membership of ten to twelve women has been established. The group is primarily in the dynamics of middle stages (see Kurland & Salmon, 1998; and Shulman, 1999, for a discussion of the middle stages of group development), although the SAGE Women's Support group is an open group, and therefore swings between beginnings, middles, and end stages rapidly at times.

Living through an era that persecuted gay and lesbian people and discouraged women from speaking their true feelings has made personally revealing themselves a challenge for most of the women in this group. Many of the women support group members are also members of peer-led discussion groups where the group norms discourage personal sharing, so it is taking a long time to develop new norms where personal sharing is encouraged, and is indeed, expected. Additional challenges are posed by the nature of an open group wherein new members drop in and out.

We have been talking about friendships for weeks. Defining the term has proved to be a slippery objective. Marjy and Carol said friends were people "who were there for each other," Sheila and Barb experienced friendship as an emotional bond irrespective of time and deeds, and Edith, Gloria, and Joyce viewed it as a relationship that took a very long time to develop.

It was interesting to me that even though almost all of the group members lived in New York City most of their lives, and many of them have known each other for decades, there was little sense of community among them. They seemed to have developed a guarded approach to each other based on assumptions, experiences, and perceptions developed over scores of years. As group leader, I have been reflecting their desire for more meaningful friendships to them and challenging them to look at some of their contradictory perceptions. By assisting them to communicate with each other in a deeper way, I hope members of the group will see themselves in relation to each other in a new light.

In the following excerpts, I refer to myself as worker. Specific terms put forth by Middleman and Wood (1990) are used in the majority of the descriptions of the skills engaged. Frequently, more than one skill is incorporated in the worker's comment. For the purposes of analysis, the skills being employed are listed above the excerpted comments of the worker.

SESSION 1

At the close of last session Gloria said, "I realize how much baggage we have when we are older. I think that our childhoods and all the abuse and stuff we lived thru are all stuff we don't want to talk about. And the more we don't talk about it, the less we have to say." When I asked her if it was keeping her from getting close to people she said it was, but she did not want to "go there and open all that up." Since Gloria is extremely quiet and withdrawn, I took particular notice of her divulgence. In the following session, I try to bring the group back to that point.

Summarizing, Partializing Information, Preserving Continuity of Work, Giving Feedback, Checking Inferences

Worker–*We've been talking about friendship, and it has been so interesting. I want to share that I've heard the obstacles different women say are challenges to more meaningful friendships. Some of you identified fear of rejection, some are afraid the person will want too much, will ask for money, or something we don't want to or can't give. Some women said that when they started to get close to someone they found things that turned them off. Carol talked about being more critical and discriminating as she gets older, and identified being less critical as a goal of hers. Getting in relationships and not having time was mentioned as an issue as well. Gloria introduced something last week we hadn't mentioned before, which is the possibility that the baggage we carry and are unwilling to talk about gets in our way. We don't want to talk about past abuse or pain and we silence ourselves in other ways. Is that what you said, Gloria?*

Gloria–Yes. I think that we get used to keeping things to ourselves and then we don't share anything about ourselves.

Reaching for Information, Identifying Personal Goals

Worker–*It sounds like that is your struggle.*

Gloria–Yes it is.

Reaching for Information

Worker–*Do you want to say more?*

Gloria–Not really. I don't like talking about my past. Please focus on someone else.

Verbalizing Group Purpose, Validating Feelings

Worker–*I understand–it is an obstacle you identified, so it makes perfect sense it would be hard to do in the group. Remember we are here to listen if you decide you'd like to open it up.*

Terry–This group helped me clarify that I don't want any friends. I love community and sharing, and these groups are divine. But that is enough, I don't want closeness. I love having coffee but I don't have time to cultivate friendships. Period.

Edith–You are so impersonal. You need to be personal to have friends. You are so cold.

Reaching for Information, Reaching for Feelings

Worker–*Edith, it would be great if you talked about yourself. What are your thoughts and feelings about how you make friends or what you would like your friendships to be like?*

Edith–Last week I said I was looking for friends and I realize you can't look for friends, they just develop. I have people in my life that have adopted me, made me family. And I didn't have to ask for it or connive to get them to recognize my birthday. And I get gifts anyway. I send cards to people because I know they like getting them. Friendships take time to develop. That is why they are hard at our age. Time and trust. (Joyce is exclaiming yes, I agree with you, smiling approvingly)

Gloria–I agree with Edith. It takes a long time to create friendships. And we erect barriers that are harder to pull down when we get older. Like what I talked about last week. All the things that happened to us in our lives.

Reaching for Feelings

Worker–*And not being able to talk about them . . .*

Gloria–Yes. And not wanting to.

Checking Inferences, Reaching for Feelings, Getting with Feelings

Worker–*That must be very painful–keeping hard things in.*

Gloria–It becomes a way of life.

Reaching for Feeling Link

Worker–*Does anyone else feel like Gloria does?*

Rachael–Gloria, maybe you are right . . . us old women have baggage . . . friends don't come easily and neither do lovers. I might never have a lover again, or a good friend and I need to acknowledge that. I was with my partner for years and spent little energy on friends. Now I am alone and I am thinking about them. And I think I find them secondary in my life. I am not so sure of their importance. I never learned the art of developing friendships. I'll connect with people and take people's numbers and then I don't call them. And like Terry said . . . do I even want friends? How important is it really? But I have to tell you; I had a beautiful connection with someone who when we were sixteen we played music together. I just ran into her last week! She came over and we made music like when we were sixteen. It was the best time I have had in so long.

Confronting Distortion, Contradiction

Worker—*Well if it was the best time you had in so long, maybe friends are important.*

Rachael—Well the real reason I don't make friends is because maybe they are into different things than me, and when we get to know each other we won't have anything in common, and they'll think I am stupid . . .

Reaching for Information, Giving Reality Check, Confronting Distortion

Worker—*Did you find out they have different interests and did they convey that they thought you were stupid? Or is it your fear?*

Rachael—My fear . . . yes . . . my perception. I know it is about my self image.

Reaching for Information Links and Feeling Links, Universalizing

Worker—*Mmmmmm . . . it is something for all of us to think about . . . what stops us sometimes . . . perception versus reality. Rachael raises a good point; that self image can be an obstacle to closeness if we perceive people not liking us because we don't like ourselves. Self image . . . so powerful . . . What about other people in the group . . . ?*

Carol—Rachael—here is another story about misperceptions. I wanted to say that when I was in the bathroom Barb passed me and didn't say hi and I thought she was mad at me. It turns out she is sick. You see how we can misjudge? We think everything is about us.

Sheila—Us old folks are more suspicious than when we were young. We ask for more and give less. We worry too much. We need to lighten up.

Gloria—Rachael reminded me of a great experience I had recently and forgot about. I ran in to an old friend I haven't seen in ten years, we are into the same things, she is a Cancer and we went to this thing together and it was so nice and we didn't have to tell each other everything. We just were enjoying the time together.

Reaching for Information

Worker–*Are you seeing her again?*

Gloria–Yes–

Terry–That is great, Gloria–you see, you are making friends.

Marjy–Rachael, your story makes me want to share something that happened to me. I had a friend who I used to play music with. I would play and she would sing. (Marjy's voice starts to tremble. I don't know if I can do this, she says.)

Attending to Feelings, Verbalizing Norms

Worker–*Its okay to cry. We are here to support you.*

Marjy–We were close and she got breast cancer and was very sick. And right before she died we got together and she asked me to play this song and I did, even though I hadn't played in years. (She starts to cry) I can't do this.

Attending to Feelings, Verbalizing Norms

Worker–*Take your time, she was important to you, this is important, you can cry . . . it's okay, take your time.* (Ann echoes me and leans towards Marjy comfortingly.)

Marjy–OK. I played the whole thing beautifully. I never could play it again and I think it was my desire to do it for her that enabled me to do it. She died shortly after. I will never forget it.

Terry–What a beautiful story, Marjy. (Others chimed in echoing.)

Giving Feedback, Getting with and Validating Feelings, Scanning, Amplifying Subtle Messages

Worker–*I appreciate how hard that was and that you were willing to share that with us. Thank you for sharing it with us. It is very moving. I see tears in almost everyone's eyes.*

Marjy–I think it is amazing that I could play that one time. I never could since.

Carol–In the 20 years I have known you I never saw you emotional.

Joyce–Yeah, Marjy, you are one tough cookie. It was so great you let yourself show emotion.

Ann–I love this group, the level of intimacy we are sharing. I hope we all come every week.

Terry–This was a good group.

Ann–We owe it to Kris (the worker)

Verbalizing Norms and Purpose, Fostering Cohesiveness, Voicing Group Achievements

Worker–*No. We owe it to all of us. I think we are doing great in creating this group to be a place to share on a meaningful level. We created a process together, it wasn't just me.*

Joyce–I am glad we don't have to talk about process anymore. Remember how we used to talk endlessly about the ground rules? Ugh.

Verbalizing Norms, Voicing Group Achievements

Worker–*It is paying off. Every group has a life of its own.*

Terry–In fact every group has a soul. Durkhein said that ages ago. I think this group had a special soul from the beginning. We are really a support group.

SESSION 2

Edith–Last week after group, I was in the bathroom and when I came out no one was here. Everyone fled! And we are talking about friendships. It is all a bunch of bullshit. It is a crock of shit, no one wants to create friendships in this group. And Terry too, I am angry at her. We were walking and left the center and all of a sudden she takes off. (Ann is very empathetic, indicating to Edith she is with her.)

Redirecting Message

Worker–*Why don't you address the group?*

Terry–Yes, Kris didn't take off on you, don't yell at her.

Edith–Well I think everyone is all talk . . . "blah blah blah" about friendship. Hah. And Terry every time, running away. . .

Terry–I said goodbye–I told you I like to walk alone. Everyone knows I am like this.

(Marjy is agitated, rolling her eyes and motioning to me to move this along.)

Edith–Oh yeah, walk alone, you like to do everything alone.

Marjy–Hey, this isn't a place to work out problems between the two of you.

Summarizing, Partializing Information, Giving Feedback, Referring to Purpose, Encouraging Group Responsibility for Process

Worker–*There are a few things happening here. Edith just expressed a lot of anger directly to the group and I want to give everyone who is anxious to talk the opportunity to respond. I would like to point out that the issue of the group leaving Edith and the dynamics of her and Terry's relationship are separate; at the same time, Terry's leaving after the group left would provoke feelings about desertion. Edith, you felt deserted twice in ten minutes! The third issue on the table is whether the group is a place to talk about interpersonal relationships.*

Use of Authority, Choosing Format, Scanning

Worker–*Jo Ann and Barb are all raising their hands to talk–looks like there's a lot of feelings opened up here. This is important and that we should hear each other out.*

Jo Ann–Edith, you can't just come into the group and expect everyone to be friends. Friendships are very rare and take a long time to cultivate. You can't just expect each person in the group to want to be friends right off the bat. It doesn't work that way.

Edith–I have known Terry for years and she is still avoiding me.

Jo Ann–I don't want to listen to your problems with Terry. That isn't appropriate.

Terry–That is what a support group is about. We are supposed to be real in here.

Breaking Taboo, Encouraging Direct Communication

Worker–*Edith brought a new dimension to the group. Before she came no one directly challenged anyone in the group before. I appreciate your honesty, Edith. I think the group is being more real since you came. It might not be comfortable but we are being more real.*

Marjy–Ever since Edith came into the group she has focused on Terry. They should work it out together outside of the group. Obviously your feelings are hurt by Terry, Edith. Maybe you should realize she doesn't want the same kind of relationship you want.

Edith–I don't want any relationship and I don't want anything from this group, except civility. "Good-bye Edith, see you next week." No one said anything to me after the group last week. And then Terry goes sprinting away like a marathon runner. And I am a marathon runner and couldn't keep up with her!

Reaching for Feeling Link

Worker–*Can anyone relate to what Edith is feeling?*

Barb–You know, I used to come and hang around after groups waiting to be asked to go along when people went out after group. I was never asked. It felt really bad. Then one day someone said, "how come you never go out with us after group?" I said I was never invited. They said, "You don't need a special invitation."

Partializing Issues, Summarizing, Reaching for Information

Worker–*I just want to point out that there are two issues on the table. The issue of what happens socially after groups in general and what happens in this group when people have interpersonal issues. Barb brings up another good question. How do new women, like Edith, learn about the group culture?*

Joyce–You just figure it out, that's all.

Ann–You know, we come from an era of not talking. We aren't brought up with very good communication skills. That's why we are so uncomfortable with all this . . . some of us are too shy to invite someone, and definitely too shy to invite ourselves.

Carol–Well I am very picky about who I spend my time with. I have a right to go out with whoever I want.

Terry–I have always hated the after group scene, who goes with who, who is invited. I find cliques unacceptable. It is why I don't go out after groups.

Jo Ann–What do you mean? You want everyone to go together?

Terry–Yes, I think everyone should be asked.

Jo Ann–Like I said, you don't just become friends by going to a group.

Edith–I don't want to be friends with everyone and go out like the last supper. That is not what I meant.

Gloria–Personally I like one-on-one contact.

Edith–Me too. Exactly.

Joyce–I was in a clique after the Tuesday night group, now that I think about it. We called it the clique mobile. It was funny. I try to sit between the people I find interesting. If I am stuck next to someone I don't like I usually get up and leave.

Marjy–I was a part of that group and found it very juvenile, and sorority-ish. A lot of women were hurt deeply. One old woman used to go searching for that group who would leave her and not say where they were going. She would go from one restaurant to the next, looking. It was so sad. That clique stuff is damaging. It is disgusting.

Barb–Yes I agree–it was pretty hurtful. I wasn't a part of it and I used to feel like something was wrong with me.

Joyce–but we weren't exclusive! Anyone could come!

Marjy–Sure, right. That is what a clique is. Exclusive.

Joyce–but we didn't exclude people.

Rephrasing, Confronting Distortion

Worker–*Maybe you didn't mean to, but can you hear that Marjy and Barb felt that the clique excluded people?*

Joyce–We didn't!

Ann–It doesn't matter if you didn't think so. That is how women felt about it. It hurt some of us. Period. You don't need to defend the clique.

Giving Feedback, Reaching for Feeling Link, Preserving Continuity, and Group History

Worker–*It is so interesting. Here is the issue of perception again, and the issue of rejection. The things we talked about theoretically months ago are being enacted in the group now. Remember this came up before; fear of rejection was talked about a lot. Now Edith is experiencing feeling rejected. It seems like Edith's experience is one that everyone can relate to.*

Terry–I belonged to a group once and we would all go out after. We would get so silly. I think silliness is important. You get close when you get silly. I want to share something. I realized after last group that I am very afraid of being abandoned. And that I run out of every group first, so I have control, and no one can hurt or reject me. My friend told me if I don't let myself experience pain I cannot experience joy. And I love joy. So I decided to risk it. I told myself that tonight I will not be the first to leave. (In fact she was second.)

Barb–I was scared to death when I came here. If you are shy you might not stick around. Who wants to be hurt?

Marjy–(tells a story about a birthday party after a group that only invited a select few.) That had ramifications for months. Women were mad or sad about it. A lot of women!

Giving Feedback, Reaching for Information

Worker–*This does hit home, doesn't it. I wonder–we are all so afraid of being rejected and abandoned . . . and easily hurt when we think that is happening . . . Do you think it goes back to childhood trauma? Does anyone remember the first time they felt this stuff?*

Barb–When I was a kid my parents were drunks and yelled and fought and the police were always there and I was on the street a lot. The kids on the block started calling me "Poison Ivy-Iodine." They would laugh and point and yell, "Poison Ivy-Iodine" whenever I came near them. I was only seven but I can still hear them.

Reflective Listening, Giving Feedback

Worker–*Ouch . . . and fifty some odd years later you still hear them.*

Ann–I know my first rejection. My mother was so jealous of me, and my relationship with my father. She hated me. So she would try to hurt me by being buddy-buddy with my friend, and lavishing her with love and affection. None for me. I have this memory of them walking way ahead of me. And I felt I was nothing. And I thought if I am nothing I will say nothing. And so I didn't for a long time.

Waiting for Feelings, Waiting for Information, Letting Silence Be

(There was a silence that I let grow as women digested this.)

Terry–well you are making me remember. When I was six, me and my twin were put in boarding school. Pushed out of the door. All of a sudden we were left to our own devices. And we would have to have a partner to walk with from school to the church and if you didn't have a partner it was humiliating and horrible. It meant no one wanted to be your friend. And I had to look out for my sister. I learned that if I were the leader, I would not be left alone. So I became a leader.

Barb–Me too! I did that too, become a leader.

Giving Feedback, Encouraging the Work, Reporting Own Feelings

Worker–*It is so fascinating, how we learned to protect ourselves. And what defenses we developed. You became leaders, Ann stopped talking . . . that is three group members who can remember specific childhood hurts. It is stimulating memories for me too. I'm not sure what defenses I created, do any of you know what defenses you created in response to the hurt?*

Ann–I learned to scapegoat myself. Look the lion in the mouth. I would provoke people to see the worst. Masochistic I guess.

Reaching for Information

Worker–*Can you say more?*

Ann–If I was in a Jewish camp I would say I was Christian. I don't do it anymore.

Gloria–My mother would say if abortion was legal when I was young she would have aborted me. It was hard to hear. And it didn't help that we were scattered all over the world . . . I was born in India and we moved all the time. I was alone a lot. I learned to sabotage my relationships so I wouldn't have to get close to them. I regret pushing people away, but I did.

Reaching for Information

Worker–*And now?*

Gloria–I still do it. I also sabotage myself. I always used to push my friend to get out there and I never would accept any praise myself. I was always pushing others in the spotlight. I never let myself do anything. I was never encouraged. I would say I still sabotage myself.

Scanning, Amplifying Subtle Messages

Worker–*Marjy you are nodding–it seems like you are relating to what Gloria is saying?*

Marjy–I am. I have done that too. I think I am afraid of success and sabotage myself if I get close to succeeding.

Gloria–Yes! Me too . . . so I don't succeed.

Marjy–I was always on my own too, Gloria. And I feel like my entire family abandoned me. I had to do everything for myself.

Jo Ann–My mother hated me. I always had this cleft palate. She told me she wishes she aborted me, so I know what that feels like, Gloria. Once she came after me with a knife. I was desperate for love. I would climb on my relations, my grandparents, or anyone who would let me and beg for it. It saved me actually.

Barb–Yes, I know that desperation. I left home when I was fifteen. I knew if I didn't either I would kill my mother or she would kill me. I would find families and worm my way in. Families with little kids, I would help the mother and become indispensable. And I would get some love. And as an adult I attached to my lover's family. My lover's mother treated me so special. My lover would get jealous, because her mother would cook for me special. Ann–you were the friend I hated. Well not hated, but were so jealous of.

Carol–Well my mother never was physically violent. She did her violence with her mouth. She was so verbally abusive. She made me want to fail . . . I'd rather fail than succeed. I remember at my graduation I was at the top of my class and she was giving me the worst sneer. I remember my first bad rejection. My mother sent me to camp, but after it was already going for a month . . . so I was the only new kid, and was paired up with a retarded kid everyone hated. I never did fit in, was never one of the group. They all knew how to swim. Not me. (Carol then tells a story about a camp counselor who tricked her into jumping off the boat after hours of Carol refusing.) I never fully trusted anyone again.

Giving Feedback, Summarizing, Voicing Group Achievements, Preserving Continuity of Work

Worker–*I'll bet trust is an issue for everyone, after all that painful stuff that happened . . . This is amazing . . . I can't believe it is after five. So much happened here today. Edith, I want to thank you again for your honesty. I think it helped us move forward. The sharing was really deep and important I think. I appreciate everyone's willingness to be vulnerable. I am sure you are all thinking about other ways you were hurt or rejected. I know I am. I think it is so awesome that people are figuring out how they adapted and the defenses they created as a result. Let's keep thinking about how we have had to respond to so much pain. I think this stuff is core to why it is hard to be intimate, and to create meaningful friendships. What a great group . . . Good work everyone . . . great personal growth work. . . . I am impressed with all of you. . . .*

Edith–I wasn't going to come back. I am so glad I did. See, Gloria–it is good to talk about these things!

ANALYSIS

As a white middle-class lesbian, I share the skin and class privilege of most of the group members. This similarity makes me especially vulnerable to countertransferences. In fact, Edith reminds me adversely of my sister, who I see as negative and difficult. I know this, so I work at staying open to Edith, and her confrontational style proves to be invaluable to the group. As a forty-nine-year-old lesbian I have suffered homophobic attacks, but the homophobia of my lifetime was not as punitive as what many of the group members have endured. I have not endured the ageist discrimination they have, and I am careful not to assume that I understand their experiences even though I share the same gender and sexual orientation.

Session One

Edith is new to the group, and her newness combined with her forthright personal and confrontational style help push the work of the group forward. Edith has a speech impediment and dresses in "corporate career style" clothes which are in contrast to other group members' casual style of dress. In these sessions she assumes the roles of deviant and scapegoat for the group (Shulman, 1999). The group is challenged, as these particular roles create uncomfortable feelings for all of us. Difficult group members are often group workers' allies. If allowed, they may show us feelings that other group members harbor and avoid, as well as provide opportunities for buried conflicts to surface (Shulman, 1999).

In this case Edith deviates from group norms by breaking taboos and directly addressing Terry, forthrightly displaying her anger about being rejected. This is threatening, as fear of rejection has been identified by several group members as a major barrier to intimacy. I immediately depersonalize the conflict, asking Edith to generalize her feelings. I am nervous because Edith is angry and I do not allow her to voice her feelings about wanting Terry's friendship. This was a missed opportunity to nurture an honest exchange of feelings. This error deprived the group of an opportunity to work through difference and expand their capability for giving mutual aid (Bernstein, 1973; Northen & Kurland, 2001; Shulman, 1999).

Social group work theorists elucidate a widely-used problem-solving process based on the work of John Dewey (Northen & Kurland, 2002, Kurland & Salmon, 1998). Diagnosing and exploring "ruptures" to the group flow is critical (Kurland & Salmon, 1998, p. 215). At times I rush or sidestep the process, as in the dynamic described above. Working through my tendency to avoid conflict is a rewarding challenge, as each time I succeed, the work of the group grows deeper. Conflict avoidance is a problem, because when a worker does not address conflict the group will avoid conflict as well, possibly feeling shame at their feelings (Bernstein, 1973).

The record shows that for a time following the above dynamic, I am responding after each expression by a group member instead of looking to the group for their responses. Most likely this stemmed from nervousness as I realize I have just made a mistake by steering Edith away from confronting Terry. "Thinking group" is essential for a group social worker (Middleman & Wood, 1990). Establishing reciprocal sharing between members is an essential element of the work and volleying responses from the worker can prevent mutual aid from occurring.

In this session Rachael questions whether friends are really important and then shares her delight in a recent encounter with an old friend. When I face her with the contradiction, she admits it is her low self-esteem that keeps her from pursuing friendships. Terry also asserts that she does not need friends, although she loves to have coffee with people, and comes to every group. These contradictions provide insight into these women's use of denial to avoid vulnerability.

Rachael's sharing opened the way for Marjy to tell a personal story that made her cry for the first time in years. Marjy's stated intent in coming to the group was feeling her feelings, and this was a great step for her and for the group. The mutual aid process was fully illuminated and engaged in this interaction, enhancing feelings of cohesiveness and intimacy for the group. Expressions of feeling and empathy embody the desired group goal of members providing mutual aid to each other (Shulman, 1999).

Session Two

I approach the following session with a "warm and fuzzy" feeling left over from the last session. I am surprised when Edith challenges the entire group in the opening go-round. She vocally expresses her anger and pain at being left by the group and then by Terry, making group members uncomfortable. Marjy responds by insisting the group is not the place for Edith and Terry to deal with their issues.

Marjy often assumes the role of gatekeeper by diverting attention to the "appropriateness" of the issue or group process. Gatekeepers try to make sure the group does not go into too deep or painful territory (Northen & Kurland, 2001; Shulman, 1999). I know it is easy for me to collude with Marjy to avoid conflict, so I deliberately ask the group for their responses after partializing the issues. Group members are angry at Edith and I show appreciation to her and name what is happening. I do so because I want her to feel supported and to demonstrate support and encouragement of direct communication.

Edith's behavior initiated an honest exchange in which women shared feelings about some members going out socially after sessions without inviting them. This work progressed and led women to share deep painful memories of early rejection in a personal way. Gloria finally disclosed some painful information about her past. It was a significant step for her. It is ironic that Edith, the instigator, was the only one who did not share an experience.

It becomes clear in the second excerpted session that early experiences of rejections left deep scars of fear and pain in the psyches of members of this group, scars that keep them from forming meaningful friendships scores of years later. The communicating they are doing with each other in the group is exciting and moving, as I can see them supporting each other in ways that bring them closer.

The practice skills that I frequently use to engage the work of the group are summarizing, partializing the issues, reaching for feelings and information, validating feelings, modeling empathy, pointing out contradictions, confronting distortions, inviting full participation, scanning, amplifying subtle messages, and verbalizing group purpose and achievements (Middleman & Wood, 1990).

Mutual aid is a cornerstone of the empowerment model of the eighties as well as a concept central to feminism. In fostering a group where peers support each other, group workers empower members by providing space, skills, and opportunities to understand and support each other. The work of assisting and enabling these old lesbians to support each other and communicate honestly and supportively enriches and expands their lives. The practice of looking to group members to collectively establish their purpose reinforces the strengths-based concepts of empowerment, and respects the "nothing about us without us" principle that old lesbian activists purport (OLOC, 1992). This strengths perspective is based in principles found in feminist, eco-systemic, wholistic, and ecological perspectives.

Incorporating a cognitive approach assists people in identifying contradictions, core beliefs, and distortions in their self-regard. I have found it helpful to encourage group members to set goals and identify their issues so they can take responsibility to change.

Next Steps

- Encourage group to continue looking at experiences that have shaped their beliefs and behavior in response to rejection.
- Work at going toward conflict and bringing differences into the open (Bernstein, 1973).
- Engage group to explore their relationships and roles, perhaps utilizing role-plays.

Group, Psychodynamic, and Sociocultural Concepts Used

Two streams of literature engaged in the work with old lesbians include theoretical perspectives in group work literature and the theoretical underpinnings of feminism. The value systems and conceptual foundations of both are completely compatible.

An important goal for the support group illustrated in the Record of Service was creating a bond conducive to the reciprocal support known as mutual aid. Mutual aid has been alluded to as the most important concept of group work (Northen & Kurland, 2001; Shulman, 1999; Moyse-Steinberg, 2004). Mutual aid creates the conditions in which people can support and assist one another with their personal goals. Being able to recognize and empathize with others, to listen to others as well as express one's self, and see the commonalities with other group members empowers participants to interact more effectively in their varied social milieus (Schwartz, 1971; Shulman, 1999). The empowerment that stems from reciprocal sharing challenges the patriarchal conditioning that teaches dependency on authority and individualism. This empowerment was pivotal for the women in the old lesbian support group who were overcoming hindrances created by ageism, sexism, and homophobia.

The work of feminists including Pharr (1988), Brownmiller (1975), Dworkin (1989), Davis (1981), and Lorde (1984), provide an understanding of the dynamics of sexism, racism and other oppressions. Their works illustrate how a paradigm of privilege and power-over has disadvantaged and disempowered women, people of color, and lesbian, gay, bisexual and transgender people. The required power sharing that the group worker must exercise in creating mutual aid groups such as the old lesbian support group contradicts the power-over paradigm and strengthens participants' sense of self-determination (Middleman, 1990; Gitterman & Shulman, 1994).

Group methodology is further empowering in its avoidance of the dependency inherent in the dyad of a patient-therapist relationship (Shaffer & Galinsky, 1989). Underlying the efficacy of group work are principles and dynamics that are antithetical to the dualistic social functioning which is the dominant culture's milieu. Group work principles of inclusion, breaking and naming taboos, mutual aid, and shattering false dichotomies are central to the power of group work, and to the success of this particular group of women (Shulman, 1999; Kurland & Salmon, 1992).

Group work also addresses the disempowerment of isolation which is a tactic of oppression, and abuse (Pharr, 1988). Participating in a group of people with similar issues can help heal the effects of internalized oppression, the learned belief of the negative messages society promulgates via stereotypes, discrimination, and slurs. Internalized oppression destroys oppressed people's self-esteem and can create negative self-fulfilling prophesies. This concept is elaborated on in the work of social theorists such as Pinderhughes (1989) and Davis (1983). In "Look Me in the Eye," Macdonald and Rich (1991) exposes the oppression that old lesbians face, and formulates a feminist analysis of ageism that incorporates an exploration of how homophobia compounds age-related discrimination, and how ageism prevents the lesbian and gay community from supporting old lesbian and gay people. Macdonald's work challenges me as a younger lesbian to examine my own beliefs about aging and old people, and my positionality in reference to them.

Positionality is the understanding of where one fits on a continuum of privilege and oppression and how one's identities affect one's relationships to those in other membership categories (Reed et al., 2000). For example, as a white, middle-class, middle-aged lesbian, I have privilege based on skin color, class and age, at the same time as being subjected to the oppressions of sexism and homophobia. To provide culturally competent services, I had to be aware of the power imbalances that are inherent within our system of hierarchies (Pinderhughes, 1989).

By participating in a group, people receive validation from others like them and self-esteem is increased (Northen, 1987). Group work bestows a sense of belonging that is central to Maslow's (1962) theory on the stages of self-actualization which posits that a sense of belonging is a universal social need.

Belonging and relating to a peer group reduces anxiety, increases self-expression, and willingness to try new ideas (Northen, 1976; Shulman, 1979). Northen (1987) attributes an improvement in members' self-esteem to the discovery that others who have the same problem are likeable.

Group work's emphasis on inclusion and validation of each person's contribution echoes concepts that are Frierian in nature, as they share an understanding of the reciprocal nature of learning and teaching, and the idea that monologue is oppressive, while dialogue is liberating (Friere, 1970). Groups such as the old lesbian support group foster the understanding that one is not alone in one's suffering by universalizing the issues members face (Shaffer & Galinsky, 1989; Northen, 1987).

Empowerment and strengths-based principles of the social work profession are fundamental in a membership perspective which conceptualizes the client's involvement as co-creators with the social worker (Falck, 1983). Empowerment is also conveyed by group work's message that each individual has something constructive to contribute (Kurland & Salmon, 1996; Dies, 1995).

A reduction of symptoms is attributed to the validation members receive in groups as well as their opportunity to ventilate (Northen, 1987; Shulman, 1999). One factor of group work contributing to its efficacy is that of breaking taboos. Social group work practitioners develop the ability to say the things people have the hardest time saying, and name the "pink elephants" in the room. At times the things that some individuals regard as shameful, deviant, or abnormal are normalized by the practitioner's ability to break taboos (Shulman, 1999). It is liberating to finally share "secrets" with the support of peers, as made evident in the sessions recorded above.

The overall goal for group participants such as this group of women is to become more effective in their lives within groups and systems to which they belong (Dies, 1995). Schwartz (1971) defines social works' function as mediating the "process thru which the individual and his society reach out to each other thru a mutual need for self-fulfillment." These objectives place group work as foundational to the social work paradigm, and were paramount with this group of old lesbians.

CONCLUSION

The task of uncovering the barriers to creating meaningful relationships is an especially significant one for old people whose circle of friends decreases with losses due to death and relocation. This is particularly true for old lesbian, gay, bisexual, and transgendered people who are isolated by homophobia in addition to ageism.

Social group work is an ideal medium for enhancing relationships and social competence as it provides a "relationship laboratory" for people (Northen & Kurland, 2001, p.73). The ROS in this article illustrates the progress that these particular group members are making in moving towards each other and engaging in meaningful exchanges of mutual aid.

Creating a ROS to view this work as a whole provided me with a model of my own practice to deconstruct and learn from, and insight into the lives and experiences of the women I work with. It was an honor and an inspiration to work with this group of old women who are bravely seeking to look at their fears and feelings, and to become closer and more vulnerable with each other. They taught me to face conflict, to be patient with the problem-solving process, to appreciate being a lesbian in the twenty-first century, and to embrace my own aging.

REFERENCES

Berkman, C., & Zinberg, G. (1997). Homophobia and heterosexism in social workers. *Social Work*, 42 (4), 319-332.

Bernstein, S. (1973). Conflict and group work. In S. Bernstein (Ed.), *Explorations in group work* (pp. 54-79). Boston: Milford House Inc.

Brownmiller, S. (1975). *Against our will: Men, women, and rape.* New York: Simon and Schuster.

Cahill, S., South, K., & Spade, J. (2000). *Outing age: Public policy issues affecting gay, lesbian, bisexual, and transgendered elders.* New York: The Policy Institute of the National Gay and Lesbian Task Force.

Davis, A. Y. (1983). *Women, race, and class.* New York: Vintage Press.

Dewey, J. (1938). *Experience and education.* New York: Macmillan. In H. Northen & R. Kurland (2001) *Social work with groups* (3rd ed., pp. 191-213). New York: Columbia University Press.

Dies, R. R. (1995). Group psychotherapies. In A. Gurman & S. Messer. (Eds.), *Essential psychotherapies: Theory and practice.* New York: The Guilford Press.

Dworkin, A. (1974). *Woman hating.* New York: Dutton.

Falck, H. (1988), *Social Work: The membership perspective.* New York: Springer.

Friere, P. (1970). *The pedagogy of the oppressed.* New York: Continuum.

Garfield, G. P., & Irizarry, C.R. (1971). The record of service: Describing social work practice. In W. Schwartz & S. Zalba (Eds.), *The practice of group work* (pp. 242-261). New York: Columbia University Press.

Garland, J., Jones, H., & Kolodny, R. (1973). A model for stages of development in social work groups. In Saul Bernstein (Ed.), *Explorations in group work* (pp. 12-51). Boston: Milford House, Inc.

Getzel, G., Kurland, R., & Salmon, R. (1987). Teaching and learning the practice of social group work: Four curriculum tools. In *Social group work, competence, and values in practice* (pp. 35-50). Binghamton, NY: The Haworth Press, Inc.

Gitterman, A. (2003). The meaning, scope, and context of the concept of social justice in social work with groups. In N. Sullivan, E. S. Mesbur, N. Lang, G. Goodman, & L. Mitchell (Eds.), *Social work with groups: Social justice through personal, community, and societal change.* Binghamton, NY: The Haworth Press, Inc.

Greene, B. (1994). Lesbian and gay sexual orientations: Implications for clinical training, practice, and research. In B. Greene & G. Herek (Eds.), *Lesbian and gay psychology: Theory, research, and clinical applications* (pp. 1-24). California: SAGE.

Kurland, R., & Salmon, R. (1998). *Teaching a methods course in social work with groups* (pp. 65-69). Alexandria, VA: Council of Social Work Education.

Kurland, R., & Salmon, R. (1992). Group work vs. casework in a group: Principles and implications for teaching and practice. *Social Work with Groups*, 15 (4).

Lorde, A. (1984). *Sister outsider*. Trumansberg, NY: The Crossing Press.

Macdonald, B., & Rich, C. (1991). *Look me in the eye: Old women, aging, and ageism*. San Francisco, CA: Spinster Books.

Maslow, A. H. (1962). *Toward a psychology of being*. Princeton, NJ: Van Nostrand.

Middleman, R., & Wood, G. G. (1990). *Skills for direct practice in social work*. New York: Columbia University Press.

Moyse-Steinberg, D. (2004). *The mutual-aid approach to working with groups: Helping people in groups learn to work better together and help each other!* New York: The Haworth Press. Inc.

Northen, H. (1987). Selection of groups as the preferred modality of practice. In J. Lassner, K. Powell, & E. Finnegan (Eds.), *Social group work: Competence and values in practice*. Binghamton, NY: The Haworth Press, Inc.

Northen, H., & Kurland, R. (2001). *Social work with groups*, 3rd ed. New York: Columbia University Press.

Old Lesbians Organizing for Change (1992). *The facilitator's handbook: Confronting ageism for lesbians 60 and over*. Houston, TX.

Pharr, S. (1988). *Homophobia: A weapon of sexism*. California: Chardon Press.

Pinderhughes, E. (1989). *Understanding race, ethnicity, & power: The key to efficacy in clinical practice*. New York: The Free Press.

Pollio, D. (2002). The evidence-based group worker. *Social Work with Groups: A Journal of Community and Clinical Practice*. Vol. 25 (4), 57-68.

Reed, B. G., Newman, P. A., Suarez, Z. E., & Lewis, E. A. (1997). Interpersonal practice beyond diversity and toward social justice: The importance of critical consciousness. In Charles D. Garvin, & Brett A. Seabury. *Interpersonal practice in social work: Promoting competence and social justice* (pp. 46-78). Massachusetts: Allyn & Bacon.

Reid, K. (1999). *Social work with groups; A clinical perspective* (pp. 98-99). Pacific Grove, CA: Brooks/Cole Publishing Co.

Schwartz, W. (1971). On the use of groups in social work practice. In W. Schwartz & Z. R. Zalba (Eds.), *The practice of group work*. New York: Columbia University Press.

Shulman, L. (1999). *The skills of helping individuals, families, groups, and communities* (pp. 437-473) (4th ed.) Itasca, IL: F. E. Peacock Publishers, Inc.

Steinberg, D. M. (2002). The magic of mutual aid. *Social Work with Groups*, 25 (1/2).

Sweethearts and Sourpusses: My Year with the Elderly

Sarah Stevenson, MSW Student

SUMMARY. This article chronicles a student's field placement experience at a drop-in center for homeless senior citizens. The student confronts her own fears and misconceptions about the senior population as she creates and implements a group-work program. Relying heavily on her knowledge of group development and group dynamics, she facilitates a current events group that provides lively atmosphere for her and the members to learn and grow from one another. *[Article copies available for a fee from The Haworth Document Delivery Service: 1-800-HAWORTH. E-mail address: <docdelivery@haworthpress.com> Website: <http://www. HaworthPress.com> © 2004 by The Haworth Press, Inc. All rights reserved.]*

KEYWORDS. Homeless, drop-in center, seniors, group work, pre-group, beginnings, middles, endings, conflict, current events group

The author thanks Robert Salmon for his continued support and guidance.

At the time this article was written, the author had just finished her first year as a Group-Work student at Hunter College School of Social Work.

[Haworth co-indexing entry note]: "Sweethearts and Sourpusses: My Year with the Elderly." Stevenson, Sarah. Co-published simultaneously in *Journal of Gerontological Social Work* (The Haworth Social Work Practice Press, an imprint of The Haworth Press, Inc.) Vol. 44, No. 1/2, 2004, pp. 53-80; and: *Group Work and Aging: Issues in Practice, Research, and Education* (ed: Robert Salmon, and Roberta Graziano) The Haworth Social Work Practice Press, an imprint of The Haworth Press, Inc., 2004, pp. 53-80. Single or multiple copies of this article are available for a fee from The Haworth Document Delivery Service [1-800-HAWORTH, 9:00 a.m. - 5:00 p.m. (EST). E-mail address: docdelivery@haworthpress.com].

http://www.haworthpress.com/web/JGSW
© 2004 by The Haworth Press, Inc. All rights reserved.
Digital Object Identifier: 10.1300/J083v44n01_04

INTRODUCTION

When I was told that my first-year placement would be at a drop-in center for homeless senior citizens, I was less than thrilled. I had requested to work with the homeless, but not with seniors. I did not want to spend the next nine months of my life working with a bunch of smelly, decrepit, crabby, judgmental old fogies. Such was my gross stereotype of the elderly. At the age of 25, I had virtually no exposure to senior citizens. I was never close with my grandparents and I had never worked with any clients over the age of 60. I thought I was in for a very boring year. In addition to my initial disappointment, I was also told I would be starting my field placement at the same time as my field instructor would be starting her job. A group worker herself, in her fifties, she had been hired as the Art and Recreation Coordinator to start a group-work program with the clients. I would be her lone assistant. My apprehension grew as I wondered what I was getting myself into.

PRE-GROUP

On my first day, I walked into the center, located in the basement of a church, and was greeted by a front-desk staff who seemed overworked and underpaid. Surrounding their desk were a few clients, waiting to either use the phone or sign up to see a case manager. Their eyes fixed on me, some with an air of curiosity, others with intense suspicion. I could hear what they were silently asking themselves; "What is this small red-headed, Little Orphan Annie-looking girl doing here?" I was asking myself the same question as, no doubt, others had before me (Cohen, 2002). The center was essentially one large, rectangular room. It had a space divided off for staff cubicles, a set of computers for clients, a pool table, a conference room, and a small dining area where breakfast, lunch and dinner were served daily. But what dominated the center were about six rows of beat-up geriatric chairs and a large television that seemed to hypnotize all who watched into a state of lethargic indifference to life. I would soon learn the rules of the center, the main one being that no client could claim ownership over a chair. A client left the chair and lost the chair. As there weren't as many chairs as there were clients, it would be unfair to assign chairs to clients, especially when clients might only be there for a day or two and then disappear. So, clients who lost a precious chair would be condemned to sit on the uncomfortable plastic dining chairs or worse, have nowhere to sit at all.

Lining the walls were shelves filled with bags. The other critical rule at the center was that clients were only allowed two bags to themselves. (Imagine fitting your entire life into two measly bags!) Some tried to bend the rule by having smaller duffle bags hidden under their chairs. I was taken aback by the smell of the place, a combination of body odor, unwashed clothes, urine, alcohol, rotting food, and bad breath. It was the smell of extreme poverty and hopelessness. It was a depressing place to be.

Most drop-in centers in New York City are designed this way and this one was no exception. The center served an estimated 175 clients per year, all 55 years of age and older. The reasons for the clients becoming homeless varied; many had recently been illegally evicted or harassed out of their apartments, while others were chronically homeless. Some were substance abusers who never got clean. Others were veterans. Most people who came to the center were not turned away, even if they were drunk or high. As long as they didn't appear to be a threat to themselves or to others, and they met the age requirement, they were allowed in.

I was pretty much shell-shocked by the end of my first day, having no recollection that any of my class readings even alluded to doing social group work in a setting such as this. My field instructor had worked for a few years at another drop-in center and had in mind what we would need to do to get a program off the ground. On my second day, she said to me, "We just need to go out there and make some noise." Her plan was to turn the television off, move the chairs out of their rows into a circle and hold a group right there, in the very middle of the center, for all to see. She assured me that clients would not move out of their chairs, so we needed to bring the group to them. "I don't like to take so long to plan a group," she insisted. I had to wonder if this was the right thing to do. I'd begun to read all about the effectiveness of planning, especially how valuable it is to a worker's self-esteem in starting a group (Kurland, 1982). Right now I really needed a self-esteem boost, as I was scared to death to "make some noise" for fear of retaliation from the clients.

BEGINNINGS

Many of my fears were confirmed over the next two months. Our group schedule consisted of a visual art group in the morning and a theatre group in the afternoon. The visual art group would take place over at the dining tables, while the afternoon theatre group would be held in the center. The first few weeks were very tough, and I struggled with understanding why I was there and what I should or should not be doing. Every morning I walked to the front of the room, turned off the TV, put on some music and braced myself for the torrent of abuse. "Go away!" "Go home!" "Leave us alone!" "Why are you doing this?" Sometimes it grew into larger diatribes against me. "You think because you're young and in school you know what's best for us. Well, you don't! We can take care of ourselves just fine and much better than you ever could. And we know a helluva lot more than you do!" These speeches were usually followed by applause and cheers. I quickly realized why my very first reading assignment in group work had to do with getting comfortable as an authority figure in a group (Kurland & Salmon, 1993). I was suffering from all the problems most group-work students go through: fear of being disliked, not knowing what my role was, and generally having absolutely no idea what I was doing. I have to say, I didn't blame them for being mad at me. If I were in my seventies or eighties and homeless, with nothing left other than a broken-down chair and two overstuffed bags, why shouldn't I be allowed to sleep in my chair all day in between the afternoon news and "One Life To Live?" Why should I have to listen to music I might not like or be forced to sit through a group I'm not interested in?

My two main problems revolved around feeling that I was infringing on the clients' right to self-determination and that the purpose of the groups was off-track. It seemed as though we had imposed ourselves on these people's lives and it had resulted in World War III. I found myself trying, day after day, to convince people that these groups were important to them, making the mistake of being the dreaded saleswoman of a group (Kurland & Salmon, 1992). There was a disconnection between the purpose we had devised for the groups and the clients' actual needs. We repeatedly said that the center needed to have groups and that all the groups were designed to promote socialization, motivation and coping with life as a homeless senior. Yet I wondered if this purpose weren't so much for the clients as for us. Again, it seemed to me that we were making all the wrong moves, including a lack of consideration for what the clients really need in relation to the purpose of a group (Kurland & Salmon, 1998).

During the majority of these spats between me and clients, front-desk staff stood and watched, motionless. We not only disrupted the clients' lives but also the front-desk staff. We had significantly shifted the balance of power in the center, as most new groups tend to do (Northen & Kurland, 2001). Because of this, it appeared that we were on our own to fend for ourselves and the staff would not assist us, at least not for a while. It was the worst feeling in the world, to think that I wasn't liked by staff or by clients. And it wasn't even October yet!

The art group met from 10-11:30. Thankfully, there were some enthusiastic artists who welcomed the chance to sit quietly and sketch or paint. Now, I've never been a visual artist and have always said that I draw stick figures badly. However, task groups, I would soon learn, were not so much about mastering a skill as they were about developing a sense of community amongst members (Wright, 1999). This was a tricky business for me in the beginning because no one seemed to be socializing, and I didn't know how to get them to do so. I knew that I and the members of the group were well into the beginning stages of group development where we both were checking each other out and testing the waters of a potential relationship (Garland et al., 1973). I ended up resorting to case work in a group, going round robin, asking people how they were doing that day and not "thinking group" at all (Kurland & Salmon, 1992; Middleman & Wood, 1990). Although I knew this was wrong, it allowed me to learn a little bit about these strange people called seniors with whom I was totally unfamiliar. Mr. T sketched beautiful, life-like portraits, which he said he hadn't done for years, since serving on a submarine in WW II. Mr. P created detailed collages as a way of coping with his alcoholism. Ms. R kept making self-portraits, attempting to, as she said, redefine herself after being harassed out of her apartment. The stories were bizarre, sad, and true. I didn't quite know what to do with what they were saying. I was overwhelmed by these people who had lived whole, rich, and wonderful lives, and were now disenfranchised and destitute. I knew this was not a true group yet and that I was just scratching the surface of who these people were. Looking back, it seems now that I was doing the needs assessment during the group rather than prior to it (Kurland, 1982).

The afternoon theatre group was usually the battle royal of the day because this was when we moved the chairs. Clients became aggressive and territorial, understandably so. We told them if they didn't want to be a part of the group they could leave. They would lose their chair, though, and that would be a big problem. Even if they were to move to another part of the center, it wouldn't matter. The group was still being held in the middle of the floor. No one could really escape it. I guess that was the point; it seemed clients did not want to talk to each other unless they were forced to do so. They did not want to move unless they were forced. I couldn't help but wonder if this were the only way to motivate the senior population. Perhaps they had become so complacent that only radical change would wake them up in their old age. Again, as a result of having no previous work experience with the elderly, I felt I had no frame of reference on which to base a judgment.

The afternoon groups were called theatre groups. One addressed any number of themes, like substance abuse or advocacy, and usually it involved a role-play of some sort followed by a discussion. Another afternoon group we developed was the traditional theatre group, where we copied a script from a play and had an impromptu reading of it. All the groups started out the same. After the initial chaos of moving the chairs, we were left with only two or three people seated, and sometimes they were there only because they were the ones unwilling to give up their chairs. As the group started, my supervisor did a lot of talking and tried to engage the potential members already seated. While the group progressed in a session, more people would eventually come and sit down to listen. Or they would hear something and respond to it from wherever they were in the center. It was an unnerving and jarring atmosphere. The phone from the front desk would be ringing. Staff stationed at that location would carry on conversations. People would fall asleep and snore. Clients would be walking in and out of the center talking to each other or themselves. Sometimes a client who was drunk or high would come up, slurring his words incoherently or starting arguments. Eventually a group would take some shape and things would settle down. Still, I was confused and disoriented. I wasn't even taking on the role of a co-facilitator. Instead, I was a group member, thinking to myself how in the world any of this related to what I was learning in school.

MIDDLES

Towards the end of October, I started to try to take more of an active stance in the theatre group. Having a theatre arts background, I felt the most comfortable in doing this. Reading scenes from a script and then discussing it afterwards was almost second nature to me, and it felt like the easiest way for me to begin to get comfortable with groups on the main floor. I suggested that we use some Shakespeare, in particular *King Lear*. The play was all too fitting for this population–a king with a family and a substantial amount of wealth and power who loses it all, becomes homeless and dies alone–perfect! It was a great play, and clients loved to read it and could relate their lives to it. It was also a way for me to confront some of the myths of homeless seniors, myths I believe we all may have. Some of these seniors were people with master's degrees, who had families, had owned property, and had consistent employment their whole lives until now. They weren't "lazy winos" as so many people assume they are. Many were educated people who had made some mistakes and were paying for them. Many staff and students at school were shocked when I said I was reading *King Lear* with my clients. "They know how to read Shakespeare?" they asked in amazement. "Yes," I replied bemusedly, "They even know how to talk about it afterwards." Pretty soon, we got requests for other Shakespeare works like *Macbeth* or *Hamlet*. People began to reminisce about parts they had played when they were younger. Now, it seemed, we were getting somewhere: We were getting more clients to talk. It was the first sign that we had begun to move into the middles of group development. People began to let down their guard and allow a more intimate relationship to develop (Garland et al., 1973).

With November came Veteran's Day. As a staff, we decided to get clients together and march down to the ceremony held at Madison Square Park with a banner saying, "Homeless Vets Are Here." The day before we set up a blank piece of canvas and had clients help us decorate it with our slogan. The head of the agency jumped on the chance to invite the press down to cover it. Here was an opportunity to flex my community organizing muscles and get clients involved in the event. Some were more than enthusiastic, allowing themselves to be interviewed and photographed. Mr. S was one, and he could talk your ear off. He was full of random cultural and historical details and had served in WW II. Years later, after he was kicked out of his apartment, he lived in the park and had fond memories of "my friends, the squirrels." Mr. T, our sketch artist, was another open and welcoming client. At 83, he walked on crutches and discussed his time on the submarine. He recalled still hearing the sounds of men dying around him during a battle. Mr. S, originally from Scotland, also served in WW II. At 86 he'd had a stroke, and now he shuffled throughout the center with his left foot always catching up to his right. He also had nightmares about the war. Finally, there was Mr. L, who had fought not only in WW II but also in Korea. He was willing to talk but was the resident stick-in-the-mud. On his good days, he would smile and say to me, "Sweetheart, sweetheart! Where are we going today?" Bad days sounded like, "Leave me alone, I hate everybody." Luckily, Veteran's Day was a good day and he agreed to speak with some reporters.

We bused our feeble clients to the ceremony. I sat with them on a park bench, watching the parade of men and women in uniform march past us. Some clients had decided not to come because they were angry at being homeless and ignored by the government. Others were proud and willing to go, but there was a touch of sadness to them. Memories flooded back, including some they had chosen to forget. I watched as they struggled to get to their feet in time to salute the flag as it was hoisted in the air. I saw the longing in their eyes to march in the parade while knowing they were too slow and too weak to do so. Or maybe they were a little embarrassed. Other vets around them had medals and uniforms to flaunt, but our clients had none, probably because theirs were lost or thrown out because such keepsakes couldn't fit in either of their two bags. At my age, they were off fighting wars I had only read about. It didn't make sense to me that these old vets had become invisible in our society, ignored and forgotten. Yet here they were, still proud to say they had served and some unashamed to admit they were homeless. Something about the day had made the seniors more real to me; they had begun to seem not so strange.

Towards the end of November I had just enough confidence to start my own group. I'd heard from staff that a current events group had been done previously and was very popular. I thought this would be a great group for me to do as I was still testing the ropes as a group worker and as a young person working with the elderly. I always loved staying abreast of the news and facilitating a good political debate. I knew that with this population opinions were probably very strong and very different from mine. I was certain this would be a unique and challenging experience. I was also ready to plan a group my way, relying on much of what I'd read to guide me through the process. I began by doing some preliminary interviewing of clients throughout the center, especially the ones who had been attending the visual art group. I asked potential members if they thought it'd be a good group to start, and most of them said yes. It would be an open group, like all the groups at the center. The difference would be that I was determined to hold it in the conference room, not in the open floor. I felt I had generated enough interest so that I could get a fair number of clients involved.

I was sorely mistaken, of course. The day of my first group, it was like pulling teeth to get clients to leave their chairs and join the group. I haggled for a good 20 minutes before I got a group of seven people to attend. I came with a very specific plan in mind: We'd discuss the purpose of the group, ground rules, and then make our way into a discussion, using that day's issue of *The New York Times* as our guide. But I was already so nervous and tired from getting people into the room to begin with that I didn't stick to my guns. I was afraid if I spent too long on something they weren't interested in, they would leave. "We're all adults here, Sarah, we know what people are suppose to do in a group, we don't need to discuss rules," Mr. G said to me patronizingly. Again, I struggled with my role as an authority figure, especially since this was my own group and I so desperately wanted the members to like me. Maybe they were right, I thought. We don't really need to do this stuff. With the group in a closed room, discussion is bound to be calmer and people will be less likely to get up and leave in the middle of it, as they do with just about all of the groups we'd been running.

As usual, I was wrong yet again. Half an hour into the discussion, people started to leave. They had appointments, they were getting tired, or they were just getting annoyed with each other. At one point, someone brought up religion and went off on a religious tangent, prompting another member to say, "I thought we were going to talk about Bush!" and leave, despite my pleading for them to stay. The discussion went all over the place, and we didn't seem to stay on one topic for longer than 45 seconds. I panicked as the third person left. "I'm supposed to be providing lots of structure right now," I thought, "But where's my structure!" (Garland et al., 1973).

My second session wasn't much better. I'd made a decision to hold it at the dining tables, hoping I would get more people to come. It seemed that clients only came to any of the groups if they actually saw them happening. Otherwise they would forget the groups even existed. I was too nervous to take the chance of holding it in the conference room again. The dining tables were a good compromise, and I did get a few new members as well as some of the same ones who had come the previous week. I was firmer this time, saying that our first session had been a little scattered and we should try to be more focused. Still, I didn't go over some ground rules and I didn't revisit the purpose of the group. It was a bit more of a civilized conversation, but there were some spats and people did get up to leave, some to go to the bathroom, and another to take a shower. We eventually came to a conclusion about what our purpose should be. But I wondered about it for the next few months. We had all decided that the purpose was "to discuss current events." But I wasn't sure if this was a true purpose or merely a content-based statement (Kurland & Salmon, 1998). It would take many more sessions before we would reevaluate our purpose again.

By December, I'd started to get a few regulars and we slowly made our way out of the pre-affiliation stage into the power and control stage (Garland et al., 1973). I had begun to notice a definite change in the members' attitudes towards each other and myself. They started to be more honest and frank and were challenging me as a worker as to how

I would respond to them. It was fascinating, hearing their points of view on the ways things used to be and the way they are now. Members often told me that my generation was ruined because of single-parent families, lack of good teachers, and television. I wasn't quite sure how to take these opinions other than to acknowledge them with a nod and a, "Hmm, interesting, tell me more." Attending and Reaching for Information, seemed to be the only skills I had gained from my readings of Middleman and Wood (1990). At each session it seemed that members got increasingly aggressive and their opinions more inflammatory.

Worker: Earlier I passed out this article by George Soros, *The Bubble of American Supremacy.* What do you guys think of this?

Mr. L: The word supremacy isn't very flattering.

Mr. S: I want to know why America keeps attracting immigrants every day despite its reputation abroad right now.

Ms. C: Money.

Mr. S: I think it's because it's still considered the land of opportunity.

Mr. H: Well, what do we mean when we say immigrant? The founding fathers were immigrants. But they are also Americans. I think we are all Americans.

Mr. S: But America likes to exploit other countries.

Ms. V: I've traveled to Africa and I can tell you what I've seen. I've seen what the United States does. It takes from the poor countries for itself. It takes the resources, it takes the land, it takes the oil, it takes everything! And it leaves the countries in Africa to starve.

Mr. L: I disagree with–

Mr. D: She's right–

Mr. C: Aw man, that's exactly what this country–

Mr. S: I don't think–

Worker: Okay, okay, okay, hold on. Hold on. I think it's great that we are all feeling so passionate about this, but in this group we need to speak one at a time. Mr. C, what were you going to say?

Mr. C: America is dumb, okay? It uses all its money for other countries and does nothing to help the people here.

Mr. W: (walks over to the group) But listen, can I just say something here? America is still, *still*, the greatest country in the world (leaves the group).

Ms. C: It won't be so great as long as God isn't being made a priority.

Mr. H: Listen. Seven percent of the population controls the majority of the country's assets. Seven percent! A lot of those people in control are Jews.

(Everyone starts talking at once. John gets up and starts pacing back and forth between the group and the garbage cans at the other side of the room.)

Worker: Whoa! I think that's a loaded statement. There are plenty of people in positions of power other than Jews.

Mr. L: I don't like categorizing people like that.

Mr. C: But when people come over to this country they're categorized. It may not be right, but that's the way it is.

Worker: Let's get back to the article we were discussing earlier . . .

I was virtually lost in how to deal with these arguments and conflicts. I felt that by setting some group norms I would essentially be telling the members how to behave, and it made me feel uncomfortable. I was annoyed that I, at 25, would actually have to tell people three times my age how to behave. What's more, I was blown away by some of the racist and anti-Semitic comments that were made by members. I hadn't a clue as to how I should deal with them. My supervisor told me I should intervene immediately when I heard a racist statement, to cut them off before they go over the line and offend. My professor told me I should explore, asking the person why they felt a certain way. I wasn't doing either, I was keeping my mouth shut and hoping it would resolve itself (Roman, 2002). I was confused because this was an open group and membership changed every week. This became one of the main challenges for me in facilitating a "come one, come all" group in that everyone in the group may be at a different stage of development (Shulman, 1999). "Come one, come all" has its advantages, but all I could see were its drawbacks. I didn't know how to relate much of what happened in the group back to my readings. A conflict happened one Friday between two people. The next session, neither one of them was there. So, did I still have to explore the conflict, or did it not matter since the members may not be in the group next week? I couldn't seem to own my role as the group worker in an open group. I needed to be providing a lot of structure and guidance. I needed to be stating the purpose and the rules at every session. I needed to intervene during conflict, regardless of whether the members would be at the next session or not (Shulman, 1999; Northen & Kurland, 2001). But I was too scared to do any of it.

I think a lot of my discomfort had to do with the age difference between myself and the members. I still didn't know how to maintain control while being flexible and not condescending. I didn't even realize the extent of it until I was assigned a case. I wanted to do a little case management during my field placement, and I was given a doozy, Ms. B. At 83 she was evicted from her apartment for not paying her rent. She had lived an interesting life as a freelance journalist, married briefly, then divorced with no children or family on which to rely. She had traveled the world, living briefly in Mexico, running a hacienda there for a time before returning to New York. When she was kicked out of her apartment, all of her things were packed up and sent to a storage facility in Yonkers. She was being charged an exorbitant amount per month. She had been living in hotels until her money ran out and during the summer she ended up sleeping downtown in the winter gardens. The police eventually picked her up and brought her to the center about a month after I'd arrived there. She had participated in some groups, mostly my current events group. She would give me articles from *The New Yorker* to use for part of some discussions. She was also a somewhat crotchety, bossy old lady, the kind that I had pictured working with when I first heard this would be my placement.

After she was assigned to me, I knew that our top priority was to get her belongings out of the storage unit in Yonkers and down into a place closer in Manhattan. Having little exposure to casework, I relied on many of the skills I was learning in group work, namely that I needed to discuss a pretty clear purpose with Ms. B about each of our sessions together (Schmidt, 1969). I'd learned my lesson from my group by now. From November to December I spent many mornings with Ms. B, on the phone to other storage facilities, asking about the price of moving and storage units. Each time I would be on the phone, Ms. B felt completely free to yell into my ear, criticizing what I was saying. "No, don't tell them that! Don't say you're a social worker, they'll take advantage of you!" The person on the other line would chuckle as they heard her bruising comments. "She's not your grandmother, is she?" some would ask. I thought if this is what it was like to have a grandmother, thank God I never had one. I'd tell her the price of a move and she'd refuse to believe it. "Movers don't get paid $50 an hour, that's highway robbery!" "I know it is," I'd say, "But this is the best deal we can get you." "Oh, don't be such a Pollyanna, Sarah, you have to be tough with these people." It seemed I wasn't doing things quite the way she wanted me to. I was too sweet, too polite and, in her words, too innocent about the way the world worked. I knew it was in her nature to be so blunt with people. I'd heard her refer to other clients as "the windbag" or "the fatso" several times. I was no different, of course.

Ms. B was in a time crunch. She had to get her stuff out of her storage unit by the second week in December or else they'd charge her an additional $500, which she would not be able to pay. We'd set a date for the movers to transfer her belongings from Yonkers to a Manhattan storage unit. She was completely unsatisfied with the price of it all but had accepted that she had no other choice. The only problem was that she and I had no way to get up to Yonkers to pay her bill before the movers came. The movers were unable to give us a ride and public transportation was nowhere near the office or the unit. So, knowing it probably wasn't the best idea but also knowing that as an intern I had a little bit of leeway in terms of how much I could get away with, I borrowed the staff attorney's car and drove her up to Yonkers the day of the move. I picked her up at 7 a.m. and we drove for an hour north, listening to NPR. We didn't say much to each other, we were both terribly nervous that there would be a glitch in our plan. We made it to the office and she paid the fee, mumbling "This is absolutely ridiculous, you're all thieves!" We then headed over to the actual unit where her things were stored. There we were reunited with all of her belongings. It was a sad sight. Her possessions had been thrown haphazardly into boxes and her furniture was taped together, some of the legs on chairs or tables broken. Ms. B wanted to go through each and every box, determined to find her furs, her jewelry, and some clothes. The movers arrived and began loading her things onto the truck. I told her we would have to wait until they were unloaded into the new unit. On the drive back down to Manhattan, Ms. B talked at length about not trusting "the Blacks and Hispanics because they're so lazy." She added, "The Asians, now they are the ones who will do what the Blacks won't, a remarkable race of people." Again, just as with my group, I was dumbfounded as to what I should say about these comments, fearing another verbal lashing about my "Pollyanna" tendencies.

When we finally arrived at the new storage unit, we were able to go through her things. I spent the next two hours lifting boxes off of tall stacks, opening them up, searching through endless amounts of books and knick knacks. We recovered some of her clothes, a few coats, one pair of boots for the winter, and some fur hats. She was so frustrated and annoyed at how unorganized everything was; dishes were on top of books, antique pieces were mixed in with sheets. As we opened each box Ms. B would gasp a sigh of relief at seeing familiar items and would also shake her head agitatedly. "Those miserable bastards," she'd say to herself. I felt sorry for her and kept telling her that it must be very hard to see her things in such disarray. Was she happy that at least she had access to them now? "Well, I guess so," she said sadly but I knew she couldn't be that excited. She still had to return to the center that evening, and she couldn't take much with her, otherwise she'd go over the two-bag limit. And she'd have to start getting rid of some of her things because she couldn't afford a unit so large. Still, she thanked me at the end of the day in her own special way. As we drove back to the center she said, "Let's stop in Duane Reade." By this point, it was 5 p.m. and I was so exhausted, I obliged her. She came out with two dark chocolate Milky Ways and a box of chocolate tea biscuits. "These are for you; they are absolutely delicious," she said. "Ms. B, you don't have to do that," I protested. "You worked very hard today, and I wish I could pay you for it, so just take these," she answered. I ate one Milky Way on the subway ride home and saved the biscuits. They are still in my kitchen, a memento of the day's work and of another moment where a senior became a real person instead of a vague image.

In January, I came back from my winter break with a new outlook on my relationship with clients and with my group. A few changes had happened, thanks to my supervisor. We had painted the center bright colors of yellow, blue and red, replacing the old army green and white motif. Volunteers had come in and redecorated the conference room, turning it into a library for the clients with shelving and small tables. But the biggest change was the chairs. They had been rearranged out of the bus station lines into a rectangular/circular shape. Now groups held on the floor were easier to start. No chairs had to be moved. A sound system also had been purchased, and group members would talk into a microphone during a session. It sounded rather odd, and again, it was found almost nowhere in any of what I'd been studying, but it made all the difference in the world. If a group were going to be held on the floor, amplifying everyone's voice would really be helpful. With an older population, many people had weak voices and couldn't project loudly enough. Now, people could actually hear each other. It was also easier to get everyone to talk one at time since they would have to wait until the microphone was available.

So, I did the unthinkable. I started holding my current events group on the main floor. I guess I'd come to the decision that, ultimately, this population could best be reached if you started where they were: in their chairs, on the floor. I'd also started talking about how old I was, how I was in school, that I was learning about group work, and getting a Master's in Social Work. I said that I didn't have the answers but I had some skills and knowledge I felt could be beneficial to them, just like they had some skills and knowledge that could be beneficial to me. I stopped thinking about it as me versus them, 25 versus 75. I had to think of us as partners in this group where we'd come to exchange ideas and learn from each other. The group and I had actually arrived well into the middles of our group, and we'd given ourselves permission to express freely what we thought about each other and the world around us (Garland et al., 1973).

I started to begin every group by clearly stating the purpose, something that would soon begin to evolve. It became a fun routine for me, and I have to say that a part of me definitely enjoyed speaking into the microphone (I was, after all, an acting major in college.) "It's Friday, it's 10 a.m. and it's time for the current events group. The purpose of this group is to talk about current events, local, national, and international issues. There are two rules to this group. The first is that everyone needs to talk one at a time, no interrupting each other. The second is that we need to respect each other. You may disagree and, in fact, it's all the more fun when you do disagree, but we need to respect each other's opinions. So, what's on your mind today?" This seemed to set the stage up so much better for a lively and engaging conversation. I'd finally caught on that this was the best way to start an open group, that I needed to consider that in an open group, it will have in itself a beginning, middle, and end and I needed to acknowledge that (Northen & Kurland, 2001).

Maybe it was because I'd graduated it to the main floor, but suddenly the current events group seemed to be one of the most talked-about groups of the week. People asked when it was happening, and if they could discuss a particular topic. I think people also just loved talking politics on a microphone; it gave them a sense of power, something they had been stripped of when they'd become homeless. A couple of patterns soon developed with each discussion, the first being that race became a major theme connected to every issue we raised. I had spent so much time focusing on my age difference that I had neglected the multitude of other cultural differences between myself and the members. It made sense to me that the black men in the group saw race as an element in many major news stories. Most of them had probably lived through some of the worst moments of racism in the country and are still feeling repercussions from it. The majority of the clients at the center were older black men. Men outnumbered women almost five to one. Though the Center was definitely very diverse, with no one culture seeming to be overrepresented, most of the members of my group who attended regularly were black. In nearly every job I'd had, I was usually the only white person in the room, and I'd grown fairly comfortable with this. I suppose that was why I didn't consider it an issue. As the group progressed, I naturally knew I had to find what Kurland (2002) deemed the element of human commonality while acknowledging the racial differences. I realize now how powerful it was to move the group to the middle of the Center. Equal and easy access to a group is essential to developing a non-racist practice, and this was inevitably a step in the right direction (Brown & Mistry, 1994). Rather than having some potential members feeling shut out or unwanted, I invited full and open participation.

Out of this developed the second major pattern: incessant and persistent conflict. I started to dive into literature about conflict, hoping to find "the answer" to my dilemma of not knowing what to do (Kurland & Salmon, 1997). I had begun to figure out, firstly, how to disagree with clients without shutting them down and destroying the group's flow. I was right to trust my own gut when it told me that if clients said something offensive I couldn't just let it go. It was my responsibility to disagree; otherwise it might look like I would be agreeing and even condoning the opinion (Northen & Kurland, 2001). But, as my professor had told me, I also had to explore "the why" behind a person's opinion. And, when I did this, it was beneficial not only to me but to the whole group. People began to realize why a person had the opinion they did and that it stemmed from their personal experiences. Rather than hating each other, or even hating me, for a viewpoint, we shared our personal histories and it humanized who we were and why we thought the way we did. With this in mind, I also started to understand and differentiate between various types of conflicts that would come up in my groups. My members lived with each other and they had conflicts all the time outside of the group. It really seemed to exemplify the idea that a group's life isn't based solely on when sessions are held, but on the time in between those sessions (Northen & Kurland, 2001). I started to notice when the conflict resulted from a need to just release built-up tension, and when it was for real. I began learning how to negotiate between separating the hostility of a member from the actual conflict itself (Bernstein, 1973). The oddest thing began to happen: I began to enjoy, even look forward to the conflicts and disagreements. They became easier to deal with because I embraced them as part of the work of the group rather than derailing it. Conflict became fun.

Worker: Well, okay. Back to Iraq, has anyone heard about the latest report saying that Bush was planning to attack well before September 11th? Does this surprise anyone?

(Members shaking head no)

Worker: Do you think he's going to win the election this year?

Mr. L: I think he would lose if Hillary ran.

Mr. B: Yeah, vote for Hillary. She'll take care of him.

Worker: Are there a lot of Hillary Clinton fans here?

Ms. C: I don't like her.

Mr. S: Nor do I.

Worker: Well, Bush isn't gaining much in popularity. He recently visited Martin Luther King, Jr.'s grave and was booed.

Mr. S: I can't believe the President of the United States is being booed. He's trying to be a good citizen in visiting Dr. King's grave.

Mr. W: It's just an election year ploy to get votes.

Mr. L: He never visited before, why this year? Ah, to get votes!

Mr. W: Why do we have to keep bashing the United States? I don't like this.

Mr. C: Listen, everybody knows that the greatest President ever was Franklin Roosevelt because he started Social Security. None of you's should be saying anything different about–

Ms. R: Hoover had a hand in creating Social Security as well–(more people start talking at once).

Worker: One at a time, everybody.

Mr. F: We all know that there were only two great presidents–FDR and Ronald Reagan.

(*Very* loud groans and some shouting are heard from other members and the center as whole)

Worker: Wait a second, wait a second, let him finish and then we can respond. Everyone is entitled to their opinion.

Mr. F: Like I said, FDR and Reagan.

I started learning how to integrate the skills for dealing with conflict like focusing on the facts of an issue, validating the anger a member may feel and changing members' disagreements into comparisons (Middleman & Wood, 1990). Beyond that, I also wanted to search for what Bernstein (1973) called "something new" rather than members having to compromise their beliefs. The something new I was looking for, I think, was a safe place for people to express their viewpoints without feeling any repercussions for it. It was hard because everyone's emotions were so high, and everyone wanted to be heard at once. But the more practice I got, the better I was at helping members learn to talk one at a time and, what's more, to listen to each other.

During my spring semester, there was a lot happening in the news, and we covered it all. Voting became a major focus of attention with the Democratic primaries in full swing. In February, the agency began a voter registration drive, and clients in particular began voicing their support for or opposition to, voting. So many of them were disgruntled and disillusioned with America that they flat out refused to register, let alone vote. In contrast, other members became activists for voting. I was amazed to discover that some of the members who were the most critical of America were also the biggest proponents of voting.

Mr. W: It's a hypocrisy! Iraq didn't do anything to us.

Mr. G: Yeah.

Mr. A: Well, when Hitler was around, we went over and stopped him.

Mr. G: Listen, the Holocaust gets a lot of attention. What this country never talks about are the thousands and thousands of black slaves that were systematically killed.

Mr. P: Or the people over in Africa who've been killed.

Mr. M: What I am sick of, is this sanctimonious rhetoric that the U.S. has going. We claim to be peace-loving when we support dictators and regimes that massacre people. Now Hitler was evil and the Holocaust was evil. But more attention should be paid to other crimes of humanity. (Many group members shake heads in agreement.)

Worker: So, I have a question. Why do people vote if they feel so strongly about the hypocrisy of U.S. policies?

Mr. G: Well, the last voter registration that Peter's Place just had convinced me that I needed to vote. I been here a year and a half, and Tuesday was the first time I registered to vote in this community.

Mr. M: I guess there's still a small shred of optimism that maybe this time things will be different.

Worker: It's interesting to hear you both say that. I've gathered that you both have a lot of strong feelings against most of what the U.S. has done in the past and have been pretty vocal about it. But now you're also being vocal about why people need to vote.

Mr. G: People need to be shown why their vote counts. If you show them why and how their vote counts, they'll do it.

It was around this time that the group began to re-think our purpose. I started asking the group towards the end of each session why we kept discussing these issues and how they affected us. The voter registration drive seemed to propel the challenging of the purpose. I felt that the group was moving into more of a political action model, where we questioned what, why, and how things were happening *and* what we could do about them (Cohen & Mullender, 1999). I began to see how the group-work process is not just about promoting things like socialization within the group. It's also about promoting social change outside of the group, changing cultural patterns of society, and aiding major social movements (Newstetter, 1935). The homeless population, particularly homeless seniors, are invisible to candidates of public office. Although we never officially changed our purpose, the work of the group began to change as members and I questioned our role in society in relation to everything we discussed each week.

Things became even more interesting when some members began to write letters to all the major Democratic candidates and ask them to visit the center and speak to some potential supporters. Still, some members were unimpressed and untouched by the possibility.

Mr. W: I just want to remind everybody before we finish that there's still a possibility of Edwards' campaign visiting us here on Monday before the primary. If everyone could just write a letter, a quick letter, that we can send there so that they know we're here and want to be heard. It can be a short letter, nothing fancy, just saying you're a client here and want someone to come.

Worker: That sounds great. What? (To Mr. K and Mr. M) You're shaking your heads "no." You don't think so?

Mr. K: No, I don't need to do that.

Mr. M: I don't think it's worth it. They ain't comin' here.

Worker: I can understand your disenchantment and I don't think you're the only one here who feels that way. But I personally feel like we have to break this stereotype of homelessness that people in this country have. It may be worth it. (William and Doug shrug their shoulders)

The next week, representatives from the Edwards and Kerry campaigns did visit the day before the Super Tuesday primary. Clients asked questions of the Edwards rep in the morning, who emphasized the campaign's message of there being two Americas in this country. It resonated with the clients, more so than the afternoon representative from the Kerry campaign, who just happened to be Kerry's sister. Fewer clients asked questions of her, despite her attempts to play to the veterans in the room, stressing how her brother was a vet and wouldn't forget them. The clients didn't seem convinced, but I tried to get them to ask questions. "Ms. B," I whispered, "Why don't you ask a question?" Ms. B screwed up her face and replied, "I don't think so. I don't really like her suit." Mr. W had a similar reaction to my encouragement of questions, "You know, she looks a lot like her brother, and he's generally compared to a horse. Not flattering." There was something oddly refreshing about these comments and I couldn't help but laugh.

Aside from the question of whether to vote or not, as well as discussions about race, perhaps the most interesting topic that we brought to the table was gay marriage. From February on it seemed that every week the papers were plastered with pictures of gay couples tying the knot. Yet week after week the group and I didn't broach the subject. I knew I was still getting used to disagreeing with members and I was certain that my 25-year-old beliefs on gay marriage were quite different from theirs. Still, I knew I had to start testing the waters as the issue became front page news almost daily.

The first time I brought it up, no one really wanted to say anything. "It's too controversial," said Ms. B, with many members nodding their heads in agreement. I didn't push the issue, as there was so much else in the news to talk about. But one day, a few weeks later, it was clear to me that we couldn't avoid bringing it up as now there were gay marriages happening in Massachusetts, upstate New York, and San Francisco. As the group began I asked people, as usual, what was on their minds and no one said a word. So I took a deep breath and plunged into the deep, murky waters of what would be the liveliest of groups yet.

Worker: Okay, well, if no one has anything to raise, I do. What do you guys think of this whole gay marriage thing?

Mr. A: I don't like gays and I don't like the idea of them marrying, period.

Mr. S: God didn't make us to have sex with the same sex.

Ms. B: Well, I think homosexuality is okay as long as people don't actually act on their feelings or desires from it.

Worker: Okay. I'd like to know where you all get your viewpoints on gay marriage from. Is it from, say, your religion?

Ms. B: It's more from my spirituality.

Mr. S: My beliefs are from the Bible, and you know what? It's wrong. When a man has to bend over another man and put his—

Worker: Okay, okay, we don't have to get graphic about this. We can have a mature conversation and debate it without getting into graphic sexual details.

Mr. S: You can't handle it! That's what homosexuality is and you can't handle it. You shouldn't have brought it up if you can't handle it.

Worker: Listen, we can discuss homosexuality and gay marriage without talking about the actual sex act that gays may perform, just like we talk about straight people without discussing the actual sex act that they may perform.

Mr. S: Fine.

Ms. U: I disagree with all of you. I feel there's nothing wrong with people being in love. It's so rare when you find it that, if you do, you should hold onto it.

Mr. S: You don't know what the hell you're talking about.

Ms. U: Oh, fuck you!

Worker: Okay, we really need to keep the foul language to a minimum here and act like adults.

Ms. U: I'm sorry.

Mr. S.: Okay, okay, I know you have to say that and all. I know it's your job to stay neutral but if you could really express yourself, I know you'd agree with me.

Worker: Actually I don't. I totally believe in gay marriage, that's my opinion. I'd also like to hear why you guys don't.

By this point, about half the staff had come out onto the floor, eyes wide open, chins dropped to the floor, gasping and staring in disbelief. The expressions on their faces seemed to say, "Why the hell are you talking about this?" As the session progressed, it was pretty much me and Ms. U talking in favor of gay marriage and the rest of the clients in practically the entire center against it. Statements like, "Gay is not the way," and "This will lead to the human race dying out," were common throughout the discussion. Emotions, as usual, were high, but the group and I managed to keep it under control. When the session ended, I felt really good that I'd finally tackled this topic. I just knew it wouldn't be the last time we'd talk about it.

Two weeks later gay marriage was discussed again, and this time I didn't have to bring it up. It also seemed that some members were a bit more vocal than before.

Worker: Mr. S, I know there's another topic you wanted to bring up.

Mr. S: Yes, Sarah, there is. This nonsense with gay marriage, I mean what is going on here? This country is going crazy.

Mr. L: I don't mind the gay marriage, so long as the gays don't have kids.

Worker: Well, the counter argument to that is that there are so many kids in foster care right now without homes and that, if gays could marry and adopt, there would be more homes for those kids to go to.

Mr. L: But that's not a family.

Mr. A: I just think that gays should have the same constitutional rights as everybody else, they are citizens!

Ms. W: Why can't we just leave the gays alone? Leave them alone, let them be, let them have their own lives and don't interfere!

Ms. T: But the Bible says that gays are wrong, they are in sin.

Mr. L: Yes and if you follow the Bible you know it's wrong. The people responsible for perpetuating this idea of homosexuality are the Middle Easterners, they started it.

Worker: Mr. L., where did you get that opinion from?

Mr. L: It says so in the Bible.

Worker: It does?

Mr. L: Yes.

(General shouts from the rest of the group saying, "It doesn't say that anywhere!")

Worker: Well, I just get nervous when someone starts making generalizations about a group of people doing one specific thing. I think we need to be careful about making generalizations like that.

Mr. M: You know, I am sick and tired of these Bible thumpers picking and choosing what to read and live by from the Bible. It makes me sick! (More shouting from group.)

Worker: Okay, listen everyone, listen. I know this is a sensitive subject, especially when we bring the Bible into it, so let's try to stay calm.

Ms. A: But you all have to understand that the Bible is a pure document and we must live by it.

Mr. M: That is the biggest bunch of garbage I have ever heard; the Bible is not pure at all.

(Even more loud shouting from the group as worker begins to laugh. As she does, so do others)

Worker: Wow! This is a really interesting debate . . .

What I loved about this session was how surprised I was that more people were in favor of gay marriage. New members and old ones felt comfortable enough to express their opinions and they stuck to their guns. This exemplified how important it is for a worker to express her disagreement with members on controversial topics. This way, it allows for other members to feel that it's all right to disagree as well (Northen & Kurland, 2001). It was never my intention to turn the group into a bunch of rainbow flag wavers but I was amazed that so many of the members actually agreed with me. I guess I was set in my belief that the majority of seniors in their seventies and eighties would be appalled by gays getting married. I was happily proven wrong, once again, about another stereotype I didn't even know I had about seniors.

ENDINGS

The group, and the center as a whole, seemed to be thriving by the beginning of April. But I was headed toward the end of my time there. I started bringing up my leaving about six weeks prior to the date. The first time I said my last day would be May 14th, the response was a round of applause and shouts of "Thank God." Ouch! I was sort of dumbfounded by the response. Were they being sarcastic? Did they even care that I was leaving? I knew that endings were a bizarre time and that people might start to act in strange ways toward me and my group (Garland et al., 1973; Northen & Kurland, 2001). I'd started to think about how different things were now as opposed to when I first got there. I remember the fear and trepidation I had those first few months and the ease I felt now. Turning off the television in the morning became fairly easy. Only a few people still gave me a hard time. The art group I'd dreaded in the beginning became an effortless morning drill and conversation naturally occurred.

Mr. G: Sarah, I keep forgetting things. I forget things all the time. Some times I think I'm getting Alzheimer's.

Worker: Well, I think it's natural for you to start forgetting things here and there at your age. Does anyone else notice that they forget things more as they get older?

Mr. W: Oh Jesus yes! I can't remember a damn thing! 'Course I think it's 'cause of all the drugs I done' (laughs as does the rest of the group).

This was the mutual aid (Steinberg, 2004) I had feared I could never facilitate. Now it seemed they didn't even need me there to talk to each other.

Each time I brought up my leaving, clients seemed shocked. "Why are you going?" some would say. I'd remind them that I was an intern and this was a temporary set-up. Part of me thought that, like Mr. G, they just naturally were forgetting that I was not permanent staff. The other part of me wondered if they had forgotten on purpose because they didn't want to remember. I thought about how hard goodbyes must be for these homeless seniors. How many people in their lives did they have to say goodbye to? How much was left for them to hold on to or rely on? I felt slightly guilty for leaving, thinking that I was becoming like everyone else in their lives that may have abandoned them or forgotten them.

My last week was pretty overwhelming. On Tuesday the staff and clients surprised me with a huge cake. Some clients gave speeches for me. Friday was my last day and my last current events group. The members made me work for it, too. The group was overly boisterous and rambunctious, with about four or five fights escalating into some name-calling where I had to intervene. My supervisor and other staff said that it was obvious that the clients were sad to see me go and most likely wanted to be involved in the last group in order to show their support of me and of what I'd done. I had to be more of an authority figure since the members showed signs of regression, but this time it came easily to me and I didn't feel uncomfortable.

At the end of the day I received flowers and a huge card wrapped up like a diploma. Inside were messages from clients and some pictures from the year, including some from the Veterans Day march. A few clients had some parting words for me, bitingly honest as always:

Mr. O: All bullshitting aside, you have a great heart and I appreciate what you've done here.

Mr. A: If I run into you in a few years and see that you've become a snobby social worker, I'll knock you on your ass.

As I walked out the door, a staff member stopped me and said, "You made me gasp so many times with your group." I looked at her curiously and asked why. "I just couldn't believe some of the stuff you all ended up talking about," she said. "Neither could I!" I said, feeling proud that I'd managed to shake things up in the short time I was there. "Wasn't it great?"

CONCLUDING STATEMENT

The question I was asked the most that last day was, "Will you work with seniors again?" I had told clients honestly how I'd felt when I first knew I'd be working with them: the sense of dread and unhappiness. Then I told them how much they had changed my mind. Sure, some of them were those crabby, smelly, and overly opinionated sourpusses I was afraid to work with. But they were also kind, intelligent, supportive, funny, and anything but boring. Before I came to the Center, had I had the choice to work with seniors or not, I'm almost certain I would have said no immediately. Now, if the choice presented itself again, I'd remember my year with these seniors and wonder if I have found the population to make my life's vocation.

REFERENCES

Bernstein, S. (1973). "Conflict and Group Work," *Explorations in Group Work*. Boston: Milford House, Inc., pp. 54-80.

Brown, A., & Mistry, T. (1994). "Group work with 'Mixed Membership' Groups: Issues of Race and Gender," *Social Work with Groups*, Vol. 17, No. 3, The Haworth Press, Inc., pp. 5-21.

Cohen, M.B. (2002). "A Tale of Transformation: How I Became a Group Worker," *Social Work with Groups*, Vol. 25 No.1/2, The Haworth Press, Inc., pp. 15-22.

Cohen, M., & Mullender, A. (1999). "The Personal in the Political: Exploring the Group Work Continuum from Individual to Social Change Goals," *Social Work with Groups*, Vol. 22, No. 1, The Haworth Press, Inc., pp. 13-30.

Garland, J., Jones, H., & Kolodny, R. (1973). "A Model for Stages of Development in Social Work Groups," S. Bernstein (Ed.), *Explorations in Group Work*, Boston: Milford House, pp. 17-71.

Kurland, R. (2002). "Racial Difference and Human Commonality: The Worker-Client Relationship," *Social Work with Groups*, Vol. 25, No. 1/2. The Haworth Press, Inc., pp. 113-118.

Kurland, R. (1982). *Group Formation: A Guide to the Development of Successful Groups*, in T. Kinney, & G. Loavenbruck (Eds.), United Neighborhood Centers for America, Inc. and Continuing Education Program School of Social Welfare, Nelson A. Rockefeller College of Public Affairs and Policy, State University of New York at Albany, pp. 1-20.

Kurland, R., & Salmon, R. (1992). "Self Determination: Its Use and Misuse in Group Work Practice and Graduate Education," in Fike & Rittner (Eds.), *Working From Strengths: The Essence of Group Work*, Center for Group Work Studies, Miami, FL, pp. 105-121.

Kurland, R., & Salmon, R. (1992). "Group work vs. Casework in a Group: Principles and Implications for Teaching and Practice," *Social Work with Groups*, Vol. 15, No. 4, The Haworth Press, Inc., pp. 3-14.

Kurland, R., & Salmon, R. (1997). "When Worker and Member Expectations Collide: The Dilemma of Establishing Group Norms in Conflictual Situations," in A. Alissi, & C. Mergins (Eds.), *Voices From the Field: Group Work Responds*. New York: The Haworth Press, Inc., pp. 43-54.

Kurland, R., & Salmon, R. (1998). "Purpose: A Misunderstood and Misused Keystone of Group Work Practice," *Social Work with Groups*, Vol. 21, No. 3, The Haworth Press, Inc., pp. 5-17.

Kurland R., & Salmon, R. (1993). "Not Just One of the Gang: Group Workers and Their Role as an Authority," in P. Ephross & T. Vassil (Eds.), *Social Work with Groups: Expanding Horizons*, The Haworth Press, Inc., pp. 153-169.

Middleman, R.R., & Wood, G.G. (1990). *Skills for Direct Practice in Social Work*. New York: Columbia University Press.

Northen, H., & Kurland, R. (2001). *Social Work with Groups* (3rd Ed.). New York: Columbia University Press.

Roman, C. (2002). "It Is Not Always Easy to Sit on Your Mouth," in R. Kurland, & A. Malekoff (Eds.), *Stories Celebrating Group Work. It's Not Always Easy to Sit on Your Mouth*. New York: The Haworth Press, Inc., pp. 61-65.

Schmidt, J.T. (1969). "The Use of Purpose in Casework Practice," *Social Work*, Vol. 14, No. 1, pp. 77-84.

Shulman, L. (1999). *The Skills for Helping Individuals, Families, Groups, and Communities*, 4th ed. Itasca, IL: Peacock Publishers Inc.

Steinberg, D.M. (2004). *The Mutual-Aid Approach to Working with Groups: Helping People Help Each Other*. New York: The Haworth Press, Inc.

Wright, W. (1999). "The Use of Purpose in On-Going Activity Groups: A Framework for Maximizing the Therapeutic Impact," *Social Work with Groups*, Vol. 22, No. 2/3, The Haworth Press, Inc., pp. 31-54.

The Sociocultural Reality
of the Asian Immigrant Elderly:
Implications for Group Work Practice

Irene Chung, PhD, CSW

SUMMARY. This article discusses how traditional social group work practice, with its conscious use of group activity and its non-verbal content, can serve as a culturally compatible service model to benefit the Asian American immigrant elderly. The goals and nature of group work practice are examined in the context of addressing the demands of this population's sociocultural reality. Cultural-specific constructs of psychological well-being and forms of emotion expression are examined to support this premise. A case illustration is used to supplement the discussion. *[Article copies available for a fee from The Haworth Document Delivery Service: 1-800-HAWORTH. E-mail address: <docdelivery@haworthpress.com> Website: <http://www.HaworthPress.com> © 2004 by The Haworth Press, Inc. All rights reserved.]*

KEYWORDS. Asian immigrant elderly, purpose and nature of groups

---

[Haworth co-indexing entry note]: "The Sociocultural Reality of the Asian Immigrant Elderly: Implications for Group Work Practice." Chung, Irene. Co-published simultaneously in *Journal of Gerontological Social Work* (The Haworth Social Work Practice Press, an imprint of The Haworth Press, Inc.) Vol. 44, No. 1/2, 2004, pp. 81-93; and: *Group Work and Aging: Issues in Practice, Research, and Education* (ed: Robert Salmon, and Roberta Graziano) The Haworth Social Work Practice Press, an imprint of The Haworth Press, Inc., 2004, pp. 81-93. Single or multiple copies of this article are available for a fee from The Haworth Document Delivery Service [1-800-HAWORTH, 9:00 a.m. - 5:00 p.m. (EST). E-mail address: docdelivery@haworthpress.com].

INTRODUCTION

The roots of social group work practice can be traced back to the Settlement House movement of the early twentieth century, where recreation-education activities were offered to help European immigrants of low socioeconomic backgrounds acculturate to mainstream American society. Based on the premise that program activities provide the essential medium for the group worker to facilitate the enhancement of human relations and the achievement of desirable goals among its participants, social group work distinctively recognizes the synergistic value of the verbal and the non-verbal content as the totality of the group experience (Middleman 1968).

Over the last three decades or so, the program activity aspect of social group work tended to be superseded by insight-oriented talking activity. This development has shifted the target clientele of group work practice from the general membership of society who shares common needs to individuals with specific problems and rehabilitative needs, and those who are expressive in emotionality and affect (Wilson 1976). Group work services for the elderly since then have also focused on serving those in institutional settings. In community centers for the elderly, social and recreational activities are no longer perceived as the domain of social group work, and are generally relegated to the responsibility of paraprofessionals (Toseland 1995). While these activities may serve the purpose of enhancing the support network and leisure activities of the elderly, the lack of attention to group purpose and process to address the participants' specific emotional needs has created a gap in service for many elderly populations. This is particularly relevant to the ethnic elderly populations in the United States, many of whom have varied culturally-specific ways of thinking, feeling, relating, and expressions of emotions (Consedine & Magai 2002). As a result, they often find it difficult to utilize the Western modality of talk therapy to cope with the stressors related to their immigration experiences (Ho 1986; Segal 2001; Uba 1994).

This article will discuss how the social group work modality, with its conscious use of activities and sensitivity to non-verbal content of emotional expression, can be utilized to support the Asian immigrant elderly in their adjustments to their lives in a new country.

THE ASIAN IMMIGRANT ELDERLY POPULATION

The Immigration Act of 1965 repealed the discriminatory legal provisions against emigration from Asian countries and brought about a major wave of Asian immigrants into the United States for the first time in American history. Subsequently, in the last two decades, a substantial number of Asian elderly have immigrated into the U.S. to join their adult children, making them the largest group of immigrant elderly in the country (Segal 2002). This group consists of predominantly Chinese elderly, followed by smaller groups of Japanese, Filipino, Korean, South Asian, and Vietnamese descent (Stokes, Thompson, Murphy, Gallagher-Thompson 2001). While each sub-group of immigrant elderly has its ethnic uniqueness, and retains, varying degrees of Asian cultural influences, they tend to be negatively affected by the erosion of the traditional Asian family and the role of the elderly as the respected head of the household (Segal 2001).

Sociocultural Stressors

The Asian immigrant elderly, like other minority immigrant elderly, face the dual demands of acculturation to American society and the preservation of their ethnic heritage. Kim, Kleiber, and Kropf (2001) discuss the psychological challenge for older immigrants to balance these demands when they have lived most of their lives in their countries of origin and are often equipped with less internal and external resources to adapt to the new world than younger immigrants. Changes in social and physical environments may cause disruption in the older immigrants' living arrangements and routine activities. Changes in roles, social relationships and support systems may undermine their sense of self and psychological well-being. Adaptation to these changes is often contingent on the older immigrants' ability to create a sense of continuity between their past and present lives, so that their immigration experiences are perceived as opportunities for positive change rather than total losses.

There are specific sociocultural factors that impact on the negotiation of this psychological task for the Asian immigrant elderly. On a societal level, this group tends to experience negative role status changes in the areas of employment, family relationship and community life. Declining physical strength and lack of marketable job skills often leave this population with no hope of finding gainful employment in the United States. They are also easy targets of discrimination and crime in their low-income neighborhoods due to language barriers and their distinctively different physical traits and lifestyles. Family dynamics are altered when the immigrant elderly have to depend on their children and grandchildren for financial support and assistance in negotiating with the English-speaking world (Segal 2002).

These negative changes also create cultural dissonance that further undermines the psychological well-being of these elderly. In the Asian culture, filial piety and respect for the elderly are core values that have persisted through generations, including those who have immigrated to distant countries (Segal 2001; Uba 1994). Thus the issues of loss, dependence, and marginalization faced by the Asian immigrant elderly can be experienced as an assault on their identity and self-worth in the context of the Asian culture.

Culturally Relevant Dimensions of Psychological Well-Being and Distress

Ingersoll-Dayton, Saengtienchai, Kespichayawattana, and Aungsuroch (2001) indicate that there are different constructs between the Western and the Asian concept of psychological well-being, which reflect the fundamental cultural values of the individual's sense of self in relation to others. In their research study of the elderly in Thailand, their findings indicate that the elderly's sense of psychological well-being is comprised of several dimensions in the context of their interaction with others. These dimensions include maintaining harmonious relationships, giving and receiving support, and earning respect within their familial and social network. While there may be variations in the emphasis of these dimensions among the Asian sub-groups, these constructs of well-being are consistent with the postulations of cross-cultural literature on the Asian conceptualization of selfhood. Unlike the Western view of the self, which emphasizes self-actualization and orientations toward autonomy, differentiation, and mastery over the environment, the Asian view of the self focuses on interdependence with other people and mastery of the self in adapting to the environment.

These drastic differences in orientation and values illustrate that psychological well-being is a subjective and learned cultural perception. By the same token, emotional distress is also caused by events and circumstances that are perceived as difficult and unacceptable in the individual's culture. Studies on Asian immigrant elderly indicate that circumstances that create their dependency on family members, such as poor health, lack of financial resources, and acculturation difficulties are generally perceived as major stressors (Segal 2001; Shibusawa & Mui 2001). The concept of dependency denotes an inability of the elderly to reciprocate care and support with their family members, and thus the implication that they do not deserve respect and care from others, which is a contraindication of the values and norms accorded to the elderly in the Asian culture. This collectivist orientation, along with the Asian cultural value that places a premium on perseverance and self-sacrifice, also tends to define distress in terms of relational failures rather than personal hardships and sufferings (Uba 1994). Thus it is important to note that the other implications of the aforementioned circumstances, such as pending death, personal hardships, and material deprivations are not perceived as distressful.

Expression of Emotions in the Asian Culture

As an individual's sense of psychological well-being and distress is largely defined by his cultural values, so is his form of emotion expression. Consedine and Magai (2002) discuss how emotion expressions are learned in cultural-specific forms and with different associated meanings. The emotional characteristic of the Asian culture is generally described as avoidance of verbal expression of strong emotions, as influenced by the cultural value that the individual needs to attain self-control over his feelings and desires, and maintain harmonious relationships with others (Segal 2002; Uba 1995). Thus feelings of happiness and distress are generally restrained and kept to oneself; positive feelings toward others are expressed through caring behaviors; negative thoughts and feelings regarding events and others are not expressed but dispelled through the individual's purposive attempts to engage in mental and physical activities to let go of those feelings (Chung 2003; Ingersoll-Dayton et al., 2001). These activities are, in essence, a culturally meaningful way of processing negative emotions and coping with stressful situations. However, such coping mechanisms can place a psychological burden on the individual in the face of overwhelming stressors, and research studies indicate that Asian American elderly are vulnerable to psychological distress in the form of depressive symptoms and somatization (Shibusawa & Mui 2001; Stokes et al., 2001).

In light of these reserved patterns of relational and communicational behavior, there is often a risk for practitioners to overlook the emotional needs of Asian clients. This writer believes that emotions are the driving force of human behavior, and even if they are not expressed verbally, they can still be understood and supported via activities and behavior and with appropriate sensitivity and sensibility. In this respect, social group work practice, with its emphasis on the process of human interactions and creative use of activities, has great potential in providing culturally syntonic services to Asian clients.

GROUP WORK PRACTICE
WITH THE ASIAN IMMIGRANT ELDERLY

Effective group work practice with ethnically diverse populations is predicated on providing a group experience that is relevant to the members' subjective perceptions of their needs, and their unique psychological and emotional state in the context of their cultural background and social conditions (Ho 1986). Chau (1992) points out that it is imperative that the goals and nature of group work intervention reflect an assessment of the clients' sociocultural needs and strengths and not apparent symptoms of psychological dysfunctions based on a Western frame of reference.

Group Goals

In examining the stressors that undermine the psychological well-being of the Asian immigrant elderly, it appears that the overarching group work goal should strive toward bridging the sense of cultural dissonance between their past and present identities. Toseland (1995) indicates that older adults generally use their past history to solidify their self-concept and self-esteem, drawing upon their unique backgrounds as a resource to cope with life transitions. She discusses the psychological significance for older adults to have an intact sense of the past:

> They (older adults) rely on their past to maintain a sense of self, to soothe them during difficult aspects of the transition to old age, and to give their life meaning. (p. 12)

For the Asian immigrant elderly, their sense of the past is marred by discrimination and marginalization in the new country, and multiple losses of social and familial roles as discussed in the earlier section. Thus, the dimensions of the aforementioned group goal should include restoration of their ethnic pride and ties with their country of origins, as well as validation of their strengths and accomplishments prior to their immigration. They are, in essence, important empowering strategies to repair the elderly's self-esteem and fortify their coping mechanisms. At the same time, these dimensions should be complemented by the objective of creating meaningful roles and relationships for the Asian elderly in their new environment to compensate for the multiple role losses incurred by their immigration experience.

Nature of Group Work Practice

The goals and objectives of group work practice for the Asian immigrant elderly need to be implemented in a context that is relevant to their cultural reality. Specifically, this relates to their views regarding distress and psychological well-being, as well as their coping strategies. As discussed in the preceding section on this issue, the quality of "interaction with others" is clearly central to the sense of well-being of Asian individuals, especially the elderly who adhere more to the traditional norms and values. Within this context, the Asian elderly gain satisfaction and joy from reciprocating care and concern with others, and earning respect for sharing their wisdom and knowledge.

These cultural norms are in many ways synonymous with the dynamics of the mutual aid process in groups. However, the format of sharing common concerns and supporting each other should support the Asian-specific form of emotional expression, which favors communication via activities and non-verbal behavior. In this regard, social group work, which uses "the doing activities" (Middleman 1968, p. 64) as "the vehicle through which relationships are made and the needs and interests of the group and its individual members are fulfilled" (p. 67), may serve as a culturally compatible service modality for this population.

The major tenets of social group work rest on the belief that communication in a social interactional process can be both verbal and nonverbal, and that the group worker needs to move with her group in whatever communication content the members are comfortable with. It recognizes that emotions are often expressed and exchanged through the non-verbal venue of actions, body language and silences, and that personal growth and bonding with others can take place as group members participate in the common pursuit of an activity goal (Northen 1969).

Selection of Group Activity

Middleman (1968) cautions that group activity needs to be viewed as a tool that requires deliberate selection. The careful planning of its content and structure is essential for the successful recruitment and participation of group members as well as the advancement of the group purpose.

For the Asian immigrant elderly, group activities should include a range of social, recreational, and educational content that will enhance their ethnic identity as well as strengthen their ties to the new country. Specifically, the activities should be conducive to creating a sense of psychological well-being from their psychosocial and cultural perspectives. Thus, celebrations of cultural festivities, preparations of ethnic foods, and enjoyment of ethnic music and movies should aim to create a sense of belonging, comfort, and security, and rekindle a sense of ethnic pride in their new country. Newspaper reading and discussion of current events in the home country as well as American society should focus on the creation of a sense of continuity and acceptance of disruptions that have occurred in the lives of the Asian elderly. Educational activities such as learning conversational English, utilization of community resources, nutrition, and health topics, need to promote feelings of self-sufficiency, and self-development.

Group Work Approaches

The aforementioned examples of group activity may be similar to common leisure activities offered in community centers for the ethnic elderly. However, the distinction between leisure activities and social group work lies with the group worker's skills in utilizing the program content in a disciplined and purposeful way to promote more effective psychosocial functioning of the group participants (Kim, Kleiber, & Kropf 2001; McNicoll & Christensen 1995). Middleman (1968) elucidates several crucial tasks of the group worker: the creative and flexible use of the program content; the conscious use of his/her relationship with the group members; and the facilitation of the interactional process among the group members. Implicit in the accomplishment of these tasks is the worker's ability to attune to the meanings of the non-verbal content communicated within the group activity, and intervene accordingly.

In working with the Asian immigrant elderly in activity groups, the group worker, who is generally perceived as an authority figure in the Asian culture by virtue of his/her role as the group leader, can take active steps to augment the connection between the group purpose and the concrete activity experience. The following group work interventions, based on this writer's own experience, have proven effective in complementing the non-verbal content of the group process.

Verbalization of group goals, process, and accomplishments. In articulating the purpose of the group as a means to alleviate the stressors faced by the Asian immigrant elderly, the worker offers validation of their struggles and accepts their willing participation in the group as a tacit acknowledgment of those issues. During the course of the group activity, the group worker's verbal articulation of emotions underlying the behavior and interactions of the members provides authenticity to their emotional struggles, as well as sanctions and options for the members to disclose their feelings if they choose to do so. In addition, the worker's periodic summation of her observations of the group progress and accomplishments will enhance the group member's awareness of their strengths and emotional growth.

Indirect discussion of sensitive issues. The worker can be creative in reaching for the latent emotional meanings of the group members' comments and behavior during the group activity. Timely initiation of role play, discussion of movies, and analysis of current events around issues that the Asian immigrant elderly are struggling with, can provide a culturally acceptable context for group members to feel supported around their painful life circumstances without disclosing personal details.

Worker's role within the activity. The worker can assume various roles depending on the nature of the activity, the dynamics of the interactional process, and the members' emotional needs. The offering of assistance to members in a task-oriented activity can facilitate their sense of mastery. On the other hand, being a participant and deferring the leadership role to members who possess the activity skills can enhance their sense of empowerment. In working with the Asian immigrant elderly, it is often helpful for the worker to partake in recreational activities with the members. Having worked hard all their lives and adhering to the cultural values of discipline and self-sacrifice, the Asian elderly may need support and role-modeling in incorporating the element of play and relaxation in their lives.

CASE ILLUSTRATION

Several years ago, this writer started a group at a senior citizen housing project for the Chinese immigrant elderly, with the stated purpose of helping them learn conversational English. Fifteen elderly attended the group sessions, which were held weekly for six months. In the first session, this writer clarified the purpose of the group in a context that was relevant to the sociocultural reality of the participants. She presented the group objective of learning English as a way to provide support for the participants in their efforts to be self-sufficient and acculturated to

American society. As she made some reference to the hardships and negative changes endured by the immigrant elderly, the group members expressed their acknowledgement by nodding, making eye contact with the worker and becoming quiet.

The group session usually began with the members learning some conversational English around a specific aspect of their daily lives. The worker, serving as the instructor, asked questions about the members' daily routines and living conditions to construct several key words and sentences in English as the teaching materials of the day. Oftentimes, this writer was able to elicit comments from the group members regarding their experiences of living alone. On one occasion, this writer picked the topic of learning to seek help in case of emergencies, and members proceeded to exchange stories of life-threatening situations, and shared their feelings of helplessness that were exacerbated by their physical frailty and language barrier.

After the initial instructional period by this writer, the group members were asked to work in small groups to practice their conversational English with each other. The group atmosphere usually became more informal as members lapsed into conversations among themselves. This writer generally rotated among the small groups encouraging mutual aid among the members and offering support and validation. Initially, the members held high standards of themselves, and would make self-admonishing remarks when they became distracted with socializing with each other. On those occasions, this writer would try to point out that learning takes place over a period of time, and that their lifetime of hard work has earned them the right to balance their work and play in their retirement years. Generally these comments would create an opportunity for the members to reminisce about their past work history with a sense of pride, which was reinforced by this writer's interest in hearing their stories and summarizing their accomplishments.

After a few group sessions, the members good-humoredly complained that it was difficult to learn a new language at their age. This writer responded with her observation that members seemed to have benefited from the group experience in other ways. She pointed out that members seemed to enjoy each other's company, and their comfort with sharing some personal stories created a familial atmosphere in the group. The members agreed with the observation, and acknowledged that it was valuable to continue attending the group despite the lack of significant progress in their conversational English.

While the group members never gave up on learning conversational English, this worker's reference to the progress of the underlying group purpose, i.e., providing emotional support to the group members, created more sanction for the members to interact with each other, and disclose personal concerns.

Several months after the group started, the bonding of the group members culminated in their positive response to this writer's suggestion that the group would celebrate the advent of Chinese New Year. As befitting the Chinese tradition, the group decided to prepare a sweet soup of glutinous rice balls–a family tradition that celebrates togetherness–to be shared during the group meeting. Without involving their group leader, the members efficiently delegated the preparatory tasks among themselves. On the day of the meeting, which took place in the community kitchen of the housing project, the group members enthusiastically worked as a team in setting up the room and preparing the cooking ingredients. At one point, everyone participated in making the rice balls by rolling a piece of dough between their palms, and then tossing the dough into a big pot of sweet soup. The act was symbolic of invoking togetherness, harmony, and happiness in the New Year. While no significant words were exchanged, there were warm smiles and a feeling of closeness among the members as they encouraged each other to partake of more portions of the sweet soup. This writer, who purposely shared with the group that it had been many years since she last sampled the sweet rice ball soup with her family, was approached repeatedly by the group members with bowls of soup and invitations to help herself to more servings.

As the celebration progressed, the group members decided to invite other non-Asian elderly and staff who were in the building. Encouraged by this writer, the members were able to explain the tradition in their broken English and the use of gestures. The members looked extremely pleased and gratified over their ability to communicate with the guests as well as the recognition they received for their cooking.

The positive outcome of the celebration and the interaction with the non-Asian elderly set a precedent for the group to continue hosting ethnic celebratory events and initiating invitations to other elderly in the building. When the group resumed meeting after the summer, the group members were ready to accept a non-Asian worker as a replacement for this writer, as well as other ethnic elderly in the building who wish to "learn conversational English."

Discussion

The Chinese immigrant elderly's group experiences demonstrate how the purposeful use of activity could promote group members' growth in a culturally relevant format.

The instruction of conversational English was a thoughtful selection of activity that held the potential of meeting the overall goal of enhancing cultural integration, self-esteem, and mutual aid among an ethnic elderly population. Specifically, it provided a sense of continuity to the Chinese elderly's immigrant status, as well as cultural-specific meanings of psychological well-being.

The execution and development of activities within the group demonstrated the importance of using the program content to enhance the group goal as the group process evolves. Middleman (1968) attributes this to the worker's flexibility, creativity, and adaptability in making the program content "an active, changing entity . . . taking its shape from the demands of the situation in which it is used" (p. 65). Thus, the celebration of Chinese New Year and the invitation of non-Asian elderly to participate in the group were meaningful program diversions, which brought about positive outcomes that are reflective of the group goals. The members' adeptness in preparing the celebration rekindled their sense of ethnic identity and pride. The opportunity to share some task-oriented activities and work closely together cemented their sense of community and affiliation. Most significantly, the experience of hosting their ethnic celebration and offering hospitality to the non-Asian elderly greatly enhanced their sense of acceptance by the community at large.

CONCLUSION

The uniqueness and efficacy of social group work practice lie in the dual foci of verbal and non-verbal content within the group interactional process. It recognizes that communication of emotions for some groups of individuals from varied backgrounds primarily takes place through activities and action. In providing the option for group members to express themselves via culturally relevant activities, social group work practice is a valuable resource in supporting the ethnic immigrant elderly whose unique emotional needs are often overlooked.

REFERENCES

Chau, K.L. (1992). Needs assessment for group work with people of color: A conceptual formulation. In J.A. Garland (Ed.), *Group Work Reaching Out: People, Places, and Power*. New York: The Haworth Press, Inc., pp. 53-66.

Chung, I. (2003). The implications of the 9/11 attacks on the elderly in NYC Chinatown: Implications for culturally relevant services. *Journal of Gerontological Social Work 40(4)*, 37-53.

Consedine, N.S., & Magai, C. (2002). The uncharted waters of emotion: Ethnicity, trait emotion, and emotion expression in older adults. *Journal of Cross-Cultural Gerontology 17*, 71-100.

Ho, M.K. (1986). A model to evaluate group work practice with ethnic minorities. In P.H. Glasser & N.S. Mayadas (Eds.), *Group Workers at Work: Theory and Practice in the '80s*. Totowa, NJ: Rowman & Littlefield Publishers, pp. 203-210.

Ingersoll-Dayton, B., Saengtienchai, C., Kespichayawattana, J., & Aungsuroch, Y. (2001). Psychological well-being Asian style: The perspective of Thai elders. *Journal of Cross-Cultural Gerontology 16*, 283-302.

Kim, E., Kleiber, D.A., & Kropf, N. (2001). Leisure activity, ethnic preservation, and cultural integration of older Korean Americans. *Journal of Gerontological Social Work 36 (1/2)*, 107-129.

McNicoll, P., & Christensen, C.P. (1995). Making changes and making sense: Social work group with Vietnamese older people. In R. Kurland & R. Salmon (Eds.), *Group Work Practice in a Troubled Society*. New York: The Haworth Press, Inc., pp. 101-116.

Middleman, R.R. (1968). *The Non-Verbal Method in Working with Groups*. New York: Associated Press.

Northen, H. (1969). *Social Work with Groups*. New York: Columbia University Press.

Segal, U.A. (2001). *A Framework for Immigration: Asians in the United States*. New York: Columbia University Press.

Shibusawa, T., & Mui, A.C. (2001). Stress, coping, and depression among Japanese American Elders. *Journal of Gerontological Social Work, 36(1/2)*, 63-81.

Stokes, S.C., Thompson, W., Murphy, S., & Gallagher-Thompson, D. (2001). Screening for depression in immigrant Chinese-American elders: Results of a pilot study. *Journal of Gerontological Social Work, 36(1/2)*, 27-44.

Toseland, R.W. (1995). *Group Work with the Elderly and Family Caregivers*. New York: Springer Publishing Co.

Uba, L. (1994). *Asian Americans: Personality Patterns, Identity, and Mental Health*. New York: The Guilford Press.

Wilson, G. (1976). From practice to theory: A personalized history. In R.W. Roberts & H. Northen (Eds.), *Theories of Social Work with Groups*. New York: Columbia University Press, pp. 1-44.

Residential Substance Abuse Treatment for Older Adults: An Enhanced Therapeutic Community Model

Frank Guida, PhD
Arnold Unterbach, MSW
John Tavolacci, MSW
Peter Provet, PhD

SUMMARY. A review of the epidemiology of substance abuse and corollary treatment capabilities for older adults is summarized. This review demonstrates that there is a growing number of older adults with substance abuse problems, and that a majority of such adults are under-diagnosed and have little access to treatment.

Research at Odyssey House, a non-profit, substance abuse and mental health treatment agency based in New York City, where older adults have been treated since 1997 within a discrete residential unit, is reviewed. Findings identify two distinct subgroups among the older adults being treated at Odyssey House: lifelong users (become dependent on drugs during adolescence) and late-in-life users (become dependent on drugs after age 45). Treatment implications are discussed in terms of the

---

[Haworth co-indexing entry note]: "Residential Substance Abuse Treatment for Older Adults: An Enhanced Therapeutic Community Model." Guida, Frank et al. Co-published simultaneously in *Journal of Gerontological Social Work* (The Haworth Social Work Practice Press, an imprint of The Haworth Press, Inc.) Vol. 44, No. 1/2, 2004, pp. 95-109; and: *Group Work and Aging: Issues in Practice, Research, and Education* (ed: Robert Salmon, and Roberta Graziano) The Haworth Social Work Practice Press, an imprint of The Haworth Press, Inc., 2004, pp. 95-109. Single or multiple copies of this article are available for a fee from The Haworth Document Delivery Service [1-800-HAWORTH, 9:00 a.m. - 5:00 p.m. (EST). E-mail address: docdelivery@haworthpress.com].

provision of special groups, such as trauma and bereavement groups for late-in-life users; and poly-substance abuse and relapse prevention groups for the lifelong users.

The Enhanced Therapeutic Community is presented as the primary social group and treatment modality for the effective care of older adults with chemical dependence problems. The community intervention is based on the values and principles of mutual aid and self-help for individuals who are willing and able to share their common experiences while supporting and comforting each other. The Enhanced Therapeutic Community is consistent and contemporary with our social work values and methods of social work with groups today, and is an effective method for the treatment of older adults with substance abuse problems. Two case study vignettes, which mirror the research and group process, are presented. *[Article copies available for a fee from The Haworth Document Delivery Service: 1-800-HAWORTH. E-mail address: <docdelivery@haworthpress.com> Website: <http://www.HaworthPress.com> © 2004 by The Haworth Press, Inc. All rights reserved.]*

KEYWORDS. Substance abuse among older adults, group work, Enhanced Therapeutic Community

INTRODUCTION

Often, substance abuse, in the minds of many, is associated with the young and the middle-aged. In fact, it is also a major health problem among older adults. As persons grow older and live longer, the public health problem of long-lasting substance abuse increases. This article first reviews the epidemiology of substance abuse and treatment capabilities for older adults in New York State and nationwide. A description of an ElderCare residential treatment and research program is presented. Within this treatment modality the community as method intervention is described and the unique potential of group work is explored. Two case studies next illustrate the clinical impact of both the community as method and specialized group work for two distinct subgroups of older adults: lifelong users and late, in- life users. Treatment recommendations are made for frontline social workers, substance abuse counselors, gerontologists and policymakers.

EPIDEMIOLOGY OF ELDERLY DRUG ABUSE

New York State's Office of Alcoholism and Substance Abuse Services (OASAS, 2002) reports that 4.5% of the 300,000+ individuals treated for substance abuse in 2000 in state-licensed programs were 55 years and older, which are 13,500 elders. The sheer number of people who are maturing into old age means increasing numbers of elderly alcohol and drug abusers (Williams et al., 1987). The U.S. Census Bureau predicts that the United States 65+ population will be the fastest-growing age group for the next 25 years (U.S. Bureau of Census, 1996). Demographic projections indicate that the number of seniors in need of drug treatment services in New York State will grow to approximately 630,000 by the year 2025 (New York State Office for the Aging, 2002). The OASAS report calls for policy and programmatic approaches to address the 2015 need for comprehensive education, prevention, and treatment efforts including cultural (language and ethnic), gender, age, lifestyle, and other relevant considerations to accommodate the needs of the 3.7 million New Yorkers over the age of 60 (19.4% of the total population). As described by the U.S. Substance Abuse and Mental Health Services Administration (SAMHSA), alcohol and drug abuse by older adults is an "invisible epidemic," and historically, older addicts have been overlooked and underserved by the vast majority of treatment providers (SAMHSA, 1998).

Substance abuse in elderly clients is a significant public health problem that is under-recognized and under-treated (Geller et al., 1989; Curtis et al., 1989). Alcohol and drug use in this population is associated with increased risks of medical illness, injury, psychiatric disorders, and socioeconomic decline (Tarter, 1995). Estimates from community studies of substance abuse by older individuals range from 2% to 10% (Adams et al., 1996), and it is reported that as many as 17% of older adults abuse alcohol and/or prescription drugs (Center for Substance Abuse Treatment–CSAT, 1998).

Alcohol and drug use is associated with a variety of medical problems. Complications from alcohol and drug abuse, leading to hospitalization in elderly clients, include cognitive disorders (Speckens et al., 1991), subdural hematomas or hip fractures secondary to falls (Pentland et al., 1986; Clark et al., 1998), and cardiovascular, liver, gastrointestinal, and infectious diseases (Eckhardt et al., 1981). In general, a history of alcohol and/or drug abuse in elderly patients is associated with high rates of medical treatment (Moos et al., 1994), and longer hospitalizations (Ingster & Cartwright, 1995). Among elderly patients admitted to general hospitals, 30% are problem users of alcohol, sedative/hypnotics, anti-anxiety agents, and/or analgesics (McInnes & Powell, 1994; Whitcup & Miller, 1987). Older substance-abusing inpatients have mortality rates approximately 2.5 times higher than expected for this older population (Moos et al., 1994).

While longitudinal studies (Reich et al., 1988; Glynn et al., 1984) have provided evidence for stable drinking and drug abuse patterns as a person ages (life-long users), Gomberg (1995, 1982) and Williams (1984) found that alcohol consumption was not consistent across time, and that subjects may actually increase their consumption as a response to age-related stresses, such as loss of employment, widowhood or other bereavement. Hurt et al. (1988) found 41% of people age 65 and older enrolled at the Mayo Clinic alcoholism treatment program reported late-onset (over age 45) symptoms of alcoholism. Guida, Tavolacci, and Provet (2003) in a study conducted at Odyssey House found that 37% of elder clients (55 and over) residing in a drug abuse treatment program were late-in-life abusers, and suggested that enhanced interventions be employed to meet the different needs of the two groups of elderly drug abusers.

TREATMENT CAPABILITY–NATIONAL

SAMHSA (1998) found that problems with alcohol and legal prescription medication affect as many as 17% of Americans age 60 and older. The number of seniors being treated for substance abuse is relatively small (1.6 % of the more than 1 million substance abuse clients in the nation). In New York State the treatment figure has grown steadily during the past decade, nearly doubling from 8,206 in 1991 to 16,247 in 1998 (OASAS, 2002). The estimated number of people age 50 or older in need of substance abuse treatment in the United States is expected to increase from 1.7 million in 2001 to 4.4 million in 2020 (Gfroerer et al., 2003). It is estimated that the rate of treatment need among this population will increase from 2.3% in 2001 to 3.9% in 2020.

Older adults typically abuse alcohol or prescription drugs, but a disturbing minority are addicted to illicit drugs such as cocaine and heroin. Further, alcohol and drug abuse by older adults is underreported, under-diagnosed and often untreated in the elderly population (Weintraub et al., 2002). Diagnosing addiction in older adults is a difficult and inexact science, often because the older adult may prevaricate due to social stigma. For example, physicians may misdiagnose symptoms of alcoholism as depression. Reid et al. (1998) found that physicians identify fewer than 50% of elderly patients who abuse alcohol or other drugs, and fewer than half of those identified as having drug and alcohol problems are referred for substance abuse treatment (Mulinga, 1999).

In 1998 CSAT published recommended treatment protocols for substance abuse among older adults. Treatment approaches should include: age-specific group treatment that is supportive and non-confrontational and aims to rebuild the client's self-esteem, with a focus on coping with depression, loneliness, and loss, and rebuilding the client's social support network. Social work groups based specifically on a mutual aid approach are designed to achieve these results (Sternberg, 1997; Toseland, 1995). Treatment staff members should be experienced in working with older adults, and linkages should be made with medical services. The CSAT report further recommended that treatment be provided in age-specific settings, to create a culture of respect for older clients; to take a broad, holistic approach to treatment that emphasizes age-specific psychological, social, and health problems; to keep the treatment program flexible; and to adapt treatment as needed in response to client gender.

HISTORY OF ELDERCARE AT ODYSSEY HOUSE

Although there are tens of thousands of older adults in need of substance-abuse treatment in the United States, few addiction-treatment centers are designed specifically for them. Odyssey House, as part of its mission to be a leader in innovative addiction and mental health services, created the ElderCare residential track in 1997 to accommodate the care and special needs of older, addicted adults.

Consistently, what we have heard from older adult residents who have prior treatment experience is that they prematurely left former programs because they could not get along with younger peers who misunderstood them or who behaved in an aggressive manner. The ElderCare track encourages older adult residents to share life experiences with other older adults who can empathize. This enhanced therapeutic community model has resulted in a 43% completion rate (as compared with 20% of drug abuse residential clients who typically complete treatment) since its inception. Close peer relationships allow residents to feel more comfortable in group treatment, to be candid about their problems in individual counseling, and to recover from their addictions; something most would be unable to do in residential treatment programs where co-participants are younger. Elder-to-elder peer relationships are important to the recovery of older adults.

The target population in our program is drug-addicted adults, with a mean age of 60 (median 63), who reside, or are homeless, in New York. Demographically in 2002, our ElderCare clients were 89% male, 11% female, 64% African American, 30% Hispanic and 6% White. The primary substance of abuse among 33% is alcohol, 31% report heroin abuse, and 34% crack/cocaine abuse. Sixty-seven percent (67%) have not completed high school or GED prep. Seventy-one percent (71%) had prior treatment episodes. Forty-three percent (43%) have a primary medical diagnosis of hypertension, 20% are HIV+, 15% have asthma, and 10% have heart problems. The average number of children reported is four (4), and the average number of grandchildren is six (6). Only nine percent (9%) report being currently married.

ElderCare Research at Odyssey House

As mentioned previously, research at Odyssey House has identified two groups of ElderCare clients (life-long and late-in-life users) and entails the design and testing of tailored treatment interventions for both groups. The independent variable in these ongoing studies is the two elder client groups. A survey was pilot tested to identify membership in both groups. Dependent variables include the psychological outcome indicators of depression, assessed by the Beck Depression Inventory (Beck et al., 1996); state anxiety, assessed by the State-Trait Anxiety Inventory (Spielberger, 1984); and motivation for treatment, assessed by the Circumstances, Motivation and Readiness Scale (De Leon et al., 1994). Anxiety and depression are traditional correlates of substance abuse (Simpson & Brown, 1998). Motivation for treatment is highly related to treatment outcomes, especially in TC-oriented treatment (De Leon, 2000). Other typical treatment indicators reported by clients on the ElderCare Survey include: type of drug, length of stay (days), medical (number of self-reported medical consequences), number of criminal justice mandates to treatment, and number of past treatment attempts.

The instruments were administered to 68 clients enrolled at the ElderCare facility. Thirty-seven percent (37%) of clients were identified as late-in-life users (became drug dependent after age 45). Their first-use mean age was 48.1 (47.5 median). Almost all late onset users started using drugs because of a traumatic event, most often, the death/divorce of spouse or death of a significant other. Forty-five clients were identified as life-long users (became dependent on a drug during adolescence and have been using since, with some periods of interruption, mostly due to prison/jail time). Their mean first-use age was 16.5 (16 median).

Findings indicate that life-long users are predominately alcohol and heroin abusers, while late-in-life users primarily abuse crack/cocaine (Chi-Square = 13.11, p < .01). Life-long users report significantly more past treatment attempts (p < .01), and more medical consequences (p < .08) as a result of their drug use. Life-long users have also been legally referred to treatment more often than late-in-life users. A trend toward higher levels of depression among late-in-life users was detected, while no differences in anxiety levels were detected. Life-long users have higher levels of motivation for treatment, and no differences exist on length of stay between the groups, with both groups averaging 10 months in treatment. It should be noted that all seven women in the sample were classified as late-in-life users, with mean first age use of 49 (median 50). However, this small sample size precluded any statistical analyses.

The two groups of ElderCare clients (life-long users and the late-in-life users) differ as to type of primary drug, past treatment attempts, and medical consequences of drug abuse. Specialized/enhanced treatment services (such as late-in-life user only group therapy) may lead to improvement in treatment planning for the two groups of Elder-Care clients and consequent outcomes. The refinement in ElderCare treatment will be further tested in a full-scale evaluation, which will feature indicator assessments at three points in time: baseline (Time 1), program completion (Time 2), and six-months post treatment (Time 3).

TREATMENT AT ODYSSEY HOUSE– COMMUNITY AS METHOD

The group work model for older adults at Odyssey House is the enhanced therapeutic community (TC). The primary group method of treatment is the community of concerned and like-minded individuals (De Leon, 2000). This approach mirrors the core values and the methods of provision of service that are central to social work with groups; that is, the individual is effectively helped when engaged as a whole person through the mutual aid and shared experiences in a group of their peers (Northen & Kurland, 2001; Steinberg, 1997). The enhanced therapeutic community can be defined as a group of peers with common goals and values, who wish to change addictive behaviors, destructive thinking, negative perceptions of self and others, through a structured social learning environment which provides professional assistance and guidance geared towards their special needs.

The enhanced therapeutic community is designed for treating chronic relapsing disorders. It is highly structured and supportive. It is an effective treatment modality for substance abuse disorders, designed to modify antisocial behavior and enhance functioning. The program provides multiple types of therapy for a variety of problems in a consistent setting. The method is flexible and can be modified to accommodate individual treatment needs as they emerge. Organized daily activities which offer job functions, new patterns of action and interaction (including mandatory participation in the running of the facility), begin at a concrete task-oriented level and advance as far as the client's capabilities and progress in treatment permit. As with many therapeutic communities, a resident might begin with kitchen duties, yet attain a position, within several months, as a department head or coordinator, under staff supervision. New ways of relating begin with the establishment of a relationship to the program as a whole and continue to expand throughout the treatment process. In the beginning, the focus is on developing trust in the community as a safe place where the client is welcomed as a potentially constructive, valuable member. At the same time, the new client is encouraged to develop relationships to assure mutual self-help.

Constructive interdependence is fostered through community rules, which require peers to challenge each other's old, dysfunctional patterns, and reward each other's new, pro-social behaviors. The clearly defined structure of job functions creates interdependence for meeting basic needs (e.g., timely meal services, transportation and escort to outside appointments). Senior residents, in more responsible positions within the structure, function as role models and teachers. New residents quickly recognize that change is not only possible but also probable.

A major focus for staff in planning and carrying out intra-group and intergroup interventions is on fostering appropriate independence in the individual resident and healthy interdependence among residents. Emphasis is on assisting residents in their search for lifestyle solutions as they learn problem-solving skills within the group setting. The goal is for each group, and the resident community as a whole, to use mutual self-help and self-discovery to attain the greatest degree of self-determination compatible with productive, healthy functioning. The level of self-determination will vary as functional abilities are expanded. Staff provides the community and individual residents with the parameters for reality testing, delay of gratification, impulse control functions, judgment, and support. This is achieved through weekly review, reflection, education, and communication at multidisciplinary case conferences and staff seminars. At case conferences, the treatment team explores and develops the differential diagnosis of each resident as well as the most appropriate treatment interventions to meet the stated goals and objectives of each individual's treatment plan. New discoveries and understanding are shared with the residents, who in turn share this with the entire community.

This clinical model was implemented for the elders of Odyssey House in 1997, when a service needs assessment found that our older adults in treatment would benefit from and stay longer in residential treatment if they had a community of their peers who could share more of their common experiences, culture and age-appropriate issues. The service needs assessment was conducted throughout Odyssey House programs and in the community through the Eastside Council on Aging (ESCOA) service providers. This panel of provider executives found that there was a population of older adults in their care who would benefit from residential chemical dependence treatment. A system of referrals was established and within one year Odyssey House had a census of 50 older adults in residential TC treatment, which relies heavily on group work.

SPECIFIC GROUP WORK METHOD

Within the larger community group TC treatment model there exist specialty groups (between 8-15 individuals). In social work with groups there are four stages of development in the life of a group: (1) inclusion/orientation, (2) uncertainty/exploration, (3) mutuality/goal achievement, (4) separation/termination (Northen & Kurland, 2001). The results of our research identified two distinct subgroups of elderly substance abusers based on onset of use/abuse, mitigating life circumstances, and stressors contributing to psychosocial dysfunction and drugs of choice. These data and information on our client allow us to ensure better inclusion and mutuality in the development and the formation of the groups tailored to the specific needs of each subgroup. This allows for thorough pre-group planning and formation (Kurland & Salmon, 1999). As our research discovered, the late-in-life users predominately abused crack/cocaine and alcohol, following a late-in-life trauma or catastrophic event. Therefore, a treatment ramification suggests that this subgroup be included in a trauma/bereavement group, especially for the women, to address their common life experiences (Shulman, 1999). The life-long users had a wide venue of drugs of abuse, which denotes poly-substance abuse issues and treatment needs, and demands more of an emphasis on relapse prevention groups. With both subgroups of older adults, treatment emphasis was placed on developing greater ego integrity and addressing generativity vs. stagnation life-stage issues (Gitterman & Shulman, 1994). This work is based on stages of human life cycle theories postulated by Erikson (1974).

The enhanced TC, as previously defined, allows our older adults in intensive residential treatment to form a primary social group within this "greater group" or "community." There are social norms and expectations that foster the emergence within each client of the ability to accept and receive positive peer pressure and pro-social values specific to older adults. This ensures that the culture of this older adult community is enhanced with the language, values, styles, customs, music, art, literature, and history that all can identify with. Altogether this creates a powerful positive social fabric that allows for age and stage-specific growth. Personal identity is revisited and solidified within the larger group, and specific issues are addressed in the small encounter groups. ElderCare clients are then encouraged to share their experiences with younger members of the broader treatment community. Giving back to the community, especially to the younger members, becomes its own reward and is experienced as wisdom. This is a gratifying experience of a positive nature, which replaces the unhealthy gratification of the quick fix of drugs and alcohol.

CASE STUDIES

John

John R. is a bright, well-spoken, 61-year-old African American male who has used drugs since age 17. He started with marijuana and then moved to heroin at age 23, and then alcohol and cocaine in later years. John describes himself as a "functional" addict, who was able to do five bags of heroin per day while working as a waiter for 13 years. John has been arrested numerous times for selling and possessing drugs. He served two years in prison. He once spent 88 days in a hospital with hepatitis A, contracted from a dirty needle. After this experience John had an abstinent period of 12 years during which time he married and met family responsibilities. John has a number of children, both in and outside of wedlock.

John describes his childhood as very stressful. He was the oldest child in a large family with an absent father and a disciplinarian mother. His mother would blame and sometimes hit John if his siblings got into trouble, because he was the responsible role model. Although John reported receiving As in high school, he claims to have had no real social life as a teenager. Upon graduation, John ran away from his family responsibilities to join the military. Although John reported years of abstinence, he has frequently relapsed, the last time in 2000 (at age 58), when he was arrested for selling heroin, went to jail for 29 days and was remanded to treatment. John spent two years in residential treatment in the ElderCare program at Odyssey House and was recently hired as a junior counselor.

John describes group work as a key to his current recovery. He believes that treatment can only be effective if a client lets go of his defenses and opens up to treatment. He believes that group "therapy" gives a client that chance. Life-long user group treatment at Odyssey House puts individuals of similar ages and similar life experiences together, where issues of traumatic etiology and relapse prevention can be discussed openly. The client begins to accept constructive criticism from his/her peers and mentors. In the group, psychological causes (such as emotional/physical trauma in a dysfunctional family) and consequences (such as depression and anxiety) of drug addiction are explored; but also clients are exposed to the real world value system of budgeting, time management, and positive, responsible behavior, some for the first time. An important issue that surfaces in group treatment for this elder population is the tendency of some members to argue that since they only have a few years left, that they should be able to use drugs and have a good time during this final period of their lives. The group can teach these individuals the lessons of exercise to clear the mind and anger management to burn the hostile, self-hating psychic fuel that still exists with these persons in recovery. The group can also remind these clients that true integrity at an elder age comes from a sense of satisfaction or at least an attempt at reconciliation with the past.

Lori

Lori M. is a 62-year-old Hispanic/African American female who started daily use of drugs at age 45. Prior to age 45, Lori had occasionally drunk alcohol or smoked marijuana at social events. Lori came from an intact family. Her father was a police officer and her mother stayed home and raised four children. She denies any family turmoil, although occasionally her father would drink to intoxication. Lori was able to complete high school and two years of college, and worked for many years as a paralegal in a Manhattan law firm. Lori married at age 25 and had two children. She describes her life as fairly stable for the next 20 years. Although after 10 years she separated and later divorced her husband, she continued working and raising her daughters.

Lori describes her "nightmare" with drugs starting after the deaths of her oldest daughter in a car accident and her beloved brother of cancer, both in the same year. She claimed an incredible despondency and began a daily use of cocaine, which kept her "numb from the pain," but at the same time "up to complete daily tasks." Eventually she started injecting cocaine, which culminated in "my shooting an eight ball a day," three-and one-half grams of cocaine per day. All of the women in the ElderCare Program report their primary drug of abuse as crack/cocaine. By age 50, Lori had been fired from her job, was HIV+, and had been arrested numerous times for drug possession and distribution. Her treatment at Odyssey House was mandated by the criminal justice system. Lori completed 18 months of treatment, clean and sober, and is now back in her community, attending outpatient individual therapy.

Lori describes her time in the enhanced TC treatment setting as critical to her recovery. She finds her late-in-life user group especially compelling. The group consists of all ElderCare clients who began abusing drugs later in life. This group includes almost all of the female Elder-Care clients and a few males. She expressed her initial surprise that all of the group members had issues around bereavement, abandonment, or loss. Lori spoke of an incredible bonding in the group. Everyone had similar issues, which facilitated empathic responses. In the group she was able, for the first time, to see the connection between her daily drug use at age 45 and the traumatic loss of her closest family members. She is further exploring this connection in individual therapy. The group work convinced her that she was, in fact, an addict; something she had always denied, despite all the contrary evidence. Members of the group also were influential in helping her to identify triggers (emotional and/or physical instigators of use), and more importantly, in how to deal with them. Lori maintains contact with a former group member, whom she considers a mentor and role model, and they both attend a weekly NA meeting together.

CONCLUSION

Drug abuse and dependence will increase significantly among the elderly population in the United States in the coming decades. Outpatient and residential treatment capacity must grow to meet the coming demand. Odyssey House has recognized this trend for some time and has initiated a treatment model for this population, which relies on community as method, group work, as well as specific groups based on research protocols. The enhanced therapeutic community employed at Odyssey House provides for a powerful community group-based treatment intervention relying on job functions, peers role modeling positive behaviors and sanctioning manipulative addictive behaviors, and various encounter groups. It is the specialty groups, based on research to practice, which attempt to address the etiology of the individual Elder Care client's addiction as an aid to tailor group treatment. For the life-long users, the groups offer relapse prevention strategies but also realistic, practical techniques for daily living success. For late-in-life users, abandonment and loss are primary issues, with clients focusing on psychological support and aftercare role modeling as adjuncts to recovery. Social workers who provide front-line residential treatment for substance abuse among the elderly population should promote the social group work described above in the context of enhanced therapeutic community care to maximize treatment outcomes in this hard-to-serve population.

REFERENCES

Adams, W.L., Barry, K.L., & Fleming, M.F. (1996). Screening for problem drinking in older primary care patients. *Journal of the American Medical Association,* 276, 1964-1967.

Beck, A. T., Steer, R.A., & Brown, G.K. (1996). *BDI–II: Manual.* San Antonio: The Psychological Corporation.

Center for Substance Abuse Treatment (1998). *Substance abuse among older adults.* Treatment Improvement Protocol (TIP) Series, No. 26.

Clark, P., De La Pena, F., & Garcia, F.G. (1998). Risk factors for osteoporotic hip fractures. *Archives of Medical Research,* 29, 253-257.

Curtis, J.R., Geller, G., & Stokes, E.J. (1989). Characteristics, diagnosis, and treatment of alcoholism in elderly patients. *Journal of the American Geriatric Society,* 37, 310-316.

De Leon, G. (2000). *The therapeutic community: Theory, model, and method.* New York: Springer Publishing Co.

De Leon, G., Melnick, G., Kressel, D., & Jainchill, N. (1994). Circumstances, motivation, readiness and suitability (the CMRS scales): Predicting retention in therapeutic community treatment. *American Journal of Drug and Alcohol Abuse*, 20, 495-515.

Eckhardt, M.J., Harford, T.C., & Kaelber, C.T. (1981). Health hazards associated with alcohol consumption. *Journal of the American Medical Association*, 246, 648-666.

Erikson, E.H. (1974). *Dimensions of a new identity*. New York: Horton Publishing.

Geller, G., Levine, D.M., & Manon, J.A. (1989). Knowledge, attitudes, and reported practices of medical students and house staff regarding the diagnosis of alcoholism. *Journal of the American Medical Association*, 261, 3115-3120.

Gfroerer, J., Penne, M., Pemberton, M., & Folsom, R. (2003). Substance abuse treatment need among older adults in 2020: The impact of the aging baby-boom cohort. *Drug and Alcohol Dependence*, 69, 127-135.

Gitterman, A., & Shulman, L. (1994). *Mutual aid groups, vulnerable populations, and the life cycle*, 2nd Ed. New York: Columbia University Press.

Glynn, R., Bouchard, G., LoCastro, J., & Hermos, J. (1984). Changes in alcohol consumption behaviors among men in the normative aging study. *NIAAA Research Monograph 14*. Washington, DC: US Government Printing Office.

Gomberg, E.S.L. (1982). Alcohol use and problems among the elderly. National Institute on Alcohol Abuse and Alcoholism, *Special Population Issues: Alcohol and Health Monograph 4*, 262-290.

Gomberg, E.S.L. (1995). Older women and alcohol use and abuse. *Recent developments in alcoholism, volume 12: Alcoholism and women*. Gallanter, M. (Ed.). New York: Plenum Press, 61-79.

Guida, F., Tavolacci, J., & Provet, P. (2003). An ElderCare exploratory study: Life-long versus late-in-life. The American Psychological Association convention, Toronto.

Hurt, R., Finlayson, R., Morse, R., & Davis, L. (1988). Alcoholism in elderly persons: Medical aspects and prognosis of 216 inpatients. *Mayo Clinical Proceedings*, 64, 753-760.

Ingster, L.M., & Cartwright, W.S. (1995). Drug disorders and cardiovascular disease: The impact on annual hospital length of stay for the Medicare population. *American Journal of Drug and Alcohol Abuse*, 21, 93-110.

Kurland, R., & Salmon, R. (1998). *Teaching a methods course in social work with groups*. Alexandria, VA: Council on Social Work Education, Inc.

McInnes, E., & Powell, J. (1994). Drug and alcohol referrals: Are elderly substance abuse diagnoses and referrals being missed? *British Medical Journal*, 308, 444-446.

Moos, R.H., Mertens, J.R., & Brennan, P.L. (1994). Rates and predictors of four-year readmission among late, middle-aged, and older substance abuse patients. *Journal of Studies on Alcohol*, 55, 561-570.

Mulinga, J.D. (1999). Elderly people with alcohol-related problems: Where do they go? *International Journal of Geriatric Psychiatry*, 14, 564-566.

New York State Office for the Aging (2002). Demographic projections to 2025: State agencies prepare for the impact of an aging New York–White paper for discussion, analysis, and summary.

Northen, H., & Kurland, R. (2001). *Social work with groups*, 3rd Ed. New York: Columbia University Press.

Office of Alcoholism and Substance Abuse Services of New York State, Bureau of Planning and Applied Research (2002). *County resource book: Service need and utilization.*

Pentland, B., Jones, P.A., & Roy, C.W. (1986). Head injury in the elderly. *Age and Aging*, 15, 193-202.

Reich, T., Cloniger, R., & Van Eerdewegh (1988). Secular trend in the familial transmission of alcoholism. *Alcoholism: Clinical and Experimental Research*, 12, 458-464.

Reid, M.C., Tinetti, M.E., & Brown, C.J. (1998). Physician awareness of alcohol use disorders among older patients. *Journal of General Internal Medicine*, 13, 729-734.

Shulman, L. (1999). *The skills of helping individuals, families, groups and communities,* 4th Ed. Ithasca, IL: F.E. Peacock Publisher, Inc.

Simpson, D.D., & Brown, B.S. (1998). Treatment retention and follow-up outcomes in The Drug Abuse Treatment Outcome Study (DATOS). *Psychology of Addictive Behaviors*, 11, 294-307.

Speckens, A.E., Heeren, T.J., & Roojmans, H.G. (1991). Alcohol abuse among elderly patients in general hospitals. *Acta Psychiatric Scandanavia*, 83, 460-462.

Spielberger, C.D. (1984). *State-Trait Anxiety Inventory: A comprehensive bibliography.* Palo Alto, CA: Consulting Psychologists Press.

Steinberg, D. (1997). *The mutual aid approach to working with groups.* Northvale, NJ: Jason Aronson, Inc.

Substance Abuse and Mental Health Services Administration (1998). *Substance abuse among older adults: National Household Survey on Drug Abuse.*

Tarter, R.E. (1995). *Cognition, aging, and alcohol. Alcohol and aging.* Beresford, T.P., & Gomberg, E. (Eds.). New York: Oxford University Press, 82-97.

Toseland, R. (1995). *Group work with the elderly and family caregivers.* New York, NY: Springer Publishing Company, Inc., 135-207.

U.S. Bureau of Census (1996). 65+ in the United States: Current population reports. *Special Reports, No. P23-190.* Washington, DC: US Government printing Office.

Weintraub, E., Weintraub, D., Dixon, L., Delahanty, J., Gandhi, D., Cohen, A., & Hirsch, M. (2002). Geriatric patients on a substance abuse consultation service. *American Journal of Geriatric Psychiatry*, 10, 337-342.

Whitcup, S.M., & Miller, F. (1987). Unrecognized drug dependence in psychiatrically hospitalized elderly patients. *Journal of the American Geriatric Society*, 35, 297-301.

Williams, G., Stinson, F., Parker, D., Harford, T., & Noble, J. (1987). Demographic trends, alcohol abuse, 1985-1995. *Alcohol Health and Research World*, 11, 80-83.

Williams, M. (1984). Alcohol and the elderly: An overview. *Alcohol and Health Research World*, 8, 3-9.

Mutual Aid Groups for Older Persons with a Mental Illness

Timothy B. Kelly, PhD

SUMMARY. Older adults with a mental illness face many life stressors as they cope with aging and mental illness. They require extra environmental supports to successfully navigate these challenges. Mutual aid groups represent a particularly potent source of support, and this article explores some of the unique practice issues and themes associated with group work for this vulnerable population. Group beginnings, authority, and intimacy themes are highlighted. *[Article copies available for a fee from The Haworth Document Delivery Service: 1-800-HAWORTH. E-mail address: <docdelivery@haworthpress.com> Website: <http://www.HaworthPress.com> © 2004 by The Haworth Press, Inc. All rights reserved.]*

KEYWORDS. Group work, older persons with mental illness, mutual aid groups, intimacy theme, authority theme

Shortly after giving birth to her only child at 17, Jessie was diagnosed with schizophrenia and was hospitalized in a large state hospital. She spent most of her late adolescence and adulthood in this institution. When large state mental hospitals were closed she was placed in a nurs-

---

[Haworth co-indexing entry note]: "Mutual Aid Groups for Older Persons with a Mental Illness." Kelly, Timothy B. Co-published simultaneously in *Journal of Gerontological Social Work* (The Haworth Social Work Practice Press, an imprint of The Haworth Press, Inc.) Vol. 44, No. 1/2, 2004, pp. 111-126; and: *Group Work and Aging: Issues in Practice, Research, and Education* (ed: Robert Salmon, and Roberta Graziano) The Haworth Social Work Practice Press, an imprint of The Haworth Press, Inc., 2004, pp. 111-126. Single or multiple copies of this article are available for a fee from The Haworth Document Delivery Service [1-800-HAWORTH, 9:00 a.m. - 5:00 p.m. (EST). E-mail address: docdelivery@haworthpress.com].

http://www.haworthpress.com/web/JGSW
© 2004 by The Haworth Press, Inc. All rights reserved.
Digital Object Identifier: 10.1300/J083v44n01_07

ing home ill-equipped to deal with her special needs. When the nursing home closed, her daughter, now an adult, agreed to take care of her, and she began receiving community treatment.

Josh lived an erratic and eccentric life, though for many years he held numerous odd jobs, got married, and had several children. After having many family and community problems, most of his family disowned him. A decade later he came to the attention of local authorities for causing a disturbance. He was found living in his trailer home malnourished, grossly disheveled, and in a manic state. He was deemed to be a danger to himself and others and became a client of the mental health system for the first time in his mid- to late-fifties.

Mavis lived a "traditional, middle-class suburban life" complete with marriage, raising healthy children to adulthood, and stable work. After her children were adults, she and her husband divorced. After moving through the expected pain and grief of a divorce, she rebuilt her life and lived without any noticeable difficulties. Mavis later began exhibiting symptoms of bi-polar disorder, but before she received any help she had gone on many spending sprees and depleted her finances. In a period of great despair she attempted suicide and came to the attention of the mental health system. In her early sixties she was diagnosed with a mental illness for the first time.

Jessie, Josh, and Mavis illustrate the diversity found among older persons living with a mental illness. They come from varied backgrounds and have a wide range of life experiences. Yet, they all enter old age having survived varied life stressors and are faced with the dual challenge of coping with the life transitions and stressors associated with aging *and* mental illness. After a brief overview of the demographics of older people with mental illness and the life stressors they face, this article will describe how mutual aid groups can be used to help older people with mental illness cope with the numerous and synergistic challenges they will likely face.

DEMOGRAPHICS AND MENTAL ILLNESS IN OLDER PEOPLE

It is well-documented that western industrialized nations have aging populations. In fact, the aging population is growing faster than any other segment of these nations (Meeks & Hammond, 2001; Raschko, 1991; Toseland, 1995; Zarit & Zarit, 1998). Compared to younger populations, diversity is greater in aging populations as older people bring with them a huge range of lifetime experiences (Stoller & Gibson, 2000). In addition to the divergent experiences that result from differences in gender, class, race, ethnicity, sexual orientation, and chance, some older adults bring a lifetime of mental illness with them into old age. Others will have to cope with a mental illness for the first time as an older person (Kelly, 1999).

The overall rate of mental illness within aging populations is not clear as there are contradictory reports. For example, a review of the literature found rates of prevalence for psychiatric problems among older people varying from 9% to 22% (Husaini, Moore, & Cain, 1994). There is also conflicting evidence about the nature of symptomology for older people. For example, the *Diagnostic and Statistical Manual of Mental Disorders* (APA, 2000) states that personality disorders become less obvious with age, and others suggest that symptoms become worse (Rose, Soares, & Joseph, 1993). This disagreement can be found with other mental disorders as well. Regardless of the exact numbers of older people experiencing a mental illness, Zarit and Zarit (1998) are right in suggesting that the psychopathology of older people is the psychopathology of younger people. Hence it follows that the numbers of older people living with a mental illness will increase as the population continues to age, especially when considering that there is clear-cut evidence that the incidence of dementia does increase with advanced age. Yet, older people continue to be underrepresented in service utilization (Husaini, Moore, & Cain, 1994; Padgett, Burns, & Grau, 1988).

LIFE TRANSITIONS AND CHALLENGES FOR OLDER PEOPLE WITH A MENTAL ILLNESS

When working with older people with a mental illness, one must bear in mind the double jeopardy they face. First, they must cope with the biological and social challenges of aging while trying to meet their common human needs. Biological changes include decreased strength, stamina, sensory perceptions, and efficiency of the major systems of the body (Cavanaugh, 1997). Social changes may include role loss, retirement, death of loved ones, decreased economic resources, and possible dependency (Berman-Rossi, 1990; Gray & Geron, 1995; Toseland, 1995; Zarit & Zarit, 1998). The human needs include: sustaining a sense of self, having influence over their environments, maintaining social relationships, feeling useful, loved, and affirmed, and having a meaningful life (Berman-Rossi, 1990; Blankenship, Molinari, & Kunik, 1996;

Burnside & Schmidt, 1994; Lowy, 1985 & 1983; Toseland, 1995). They must attempt to meet these needs and cope with changes associated with aging while also facing the challenges with the increased risks associated with mental illness. When these physical and social changes occur in the context of a mental illness, meeting basic human needs becomes much more difficult.

Zarit and Zarit (1995) discuss the disruption in the life course that can occur for people as they experience a mental illness. A ripple effect occurs throughout the rest of their lives. For example, if someone develops schizophrenia earlier in his or her lifetime, opportunities and resources are greatly limited. When these persons reach old age, their limited social resources can become even more stretched and strained as a result of aging. If a mental illness develops for the first time in later life, they may need to make a claim on social resources at the same time these are decreasing as a result of aging. Secondly, some of the symptoms of mental illness may make it more difficult for older people and their social resources to reach out for one another.

GROUP WORK AND OLDER ADULTS
WITH A MENTAL ILLNESS

Group work is an ideal approach for helping people navigate stressful life transitions or cope with a vulnerable life condition or circumstance (Gitterman, 1994). Mutual aid groups can be an important substitute for lost social support, provide a vehicle for coping with a devastating life transition, restore diminished self-concept, prompt life review, and maximize strengths while promoting health and mental health. These benefits occur as a result of the dynamics of mutual aid described by Shulman (1999). These dynamics are sharing data, the dialectical process, entering taboo areas, the "all in the same boat" phenomenon, mutual support, mutual demand, individual problem-solving, rehearsal, and the strength-in-numbers phenomenon. The group worker uses his or her skills to develop these dynamics in the service of helping the group members work on common problems over the life of the group.

Unfortunately, it is sometimes assumed that older adults in general are unable to benefit or unwilling to participate in therapeutic services (Lagana & Shanks, 2002). Older adults with a mental illness face even greater bias. Yet, when appropriately designed group work services are provided, older adults with mental illnesses demonstrate great capacity to use and benefit from the dynamics of mutual aid as they navigate the stressful life transitions associated with aging and mental illness. The ways in which the dynamics appear may look different than when working with other populations, but the skilled group worker will recognize and be able to facilitate the power of group work for older adults living with a mental illness. Several examples of the power of mutual aid will be presented next, followed by a discussion of how beginnings and the common group work themes of intimacy and authority may look different when working with this special population.

The Power of Mutual Aid

Older people with chronic mental illness can benefit from the powerful dynamics of mutual aid. Despite members having a wide range of psychiatric disability and functional ability, members in the author's groups contributed to and benefited from participation, even the most disabled. Not all members were able to verbalize as clearly as others. Some of the more disabled members rarely participated in some of the more psychological discussions that occurred, however the structure of the day allowed all members to participate in some part of the daily activities. Activity was purposefully used in a way that would allow all members, including the less verbal, to participate in the life of the group. Interestingly, the dynamics of mutual aid slowly pulled all members into all aspects of work of the group, and everyone was able to participate in the "psychological" work at various times.

One member who suffered with almost constant auditory hallucinations was initially very withdrawn and inwardly focused. After being part of the group for several weeks, another member who also had constant auditory hallucinations but had learned to live and function with them simply said to her, "Jessie, you leave those people alone. They are not here right now and we are. You leave them alone and talk to us." The worker was amazed as Jessie joined in the discussion for a few minutes. This member, and later others, consistently made this demand for work on Jessie in a way that the worker would never have been able to do. Though never particularly verbal, Jessie became more engaged with the group and after many months would occasionally contribute to group discussions in very meaningful ways. For example, one day the group was working on the stressful relationships they had with their home providers or family members they lived with. Ella was discussing how her daughter was threatening to put her in a home again. Ella had stopped taking her medicine and was staying up through the night disturbing everyone in the household. The group was engaged in problem-solving with Ella and trying to convince her to start taking her medication again. Jessie spoke up in her very quiet whispering voice and described how her daughter threatened the same thing many months ago. Jessie reported how she could not sleep at night, would talk to her voices, and make a mess of the house. She did not want to go back into an institution, so even though she hated how the medicine made her feel, she began taking it again. She also decided to start cleaning the house and helping with the cooking to make things easier for her daughter. Jessie suggested that Ella do the same. The group was stunned by Jessie's verbal "outburst" and it made a huge impression on Ella. Ella took Jessie's advice and averted a hospitalization and placement in a care home. Thus, even one of the lower functioning members benefitted from and facilitated mutual aid.

Beginnings

To maximize the dynamics of mutual aid, attention must be paid to a group's beginning. The beginning phase of work consists of pre-group planning and the initial contacts with members and the group (Kurland, 1978; Gitterman, 1994; Shulman, 1999). In terms of pre-group planning, there is a body of literature that describes group formation for older adults. Many authors describe exclusionary criteria for group membership for older people. This list includes such things as disturbed and wandering persons, incontinent persons, persons with active psychosis or psychotic depression, persons with bipolar disorder, deaf persons, hypochondriacal persons, persons with dementia, paranoid persons, persons with bizarre or threatening behaviors, persons with very deviant behavior, and persons who are "too frail" (Altholz, Burnside 1994b; Kennedy, 2000; Lesser, Lazarus, Frankel, & Havasy, 1981; Toseland, 1995). If such a list were followed, it would be impossible to have groups for older people coping with a mental illness. Groups should be formed around a common purpose and felt need, rather than on strict selection criteria. For example, the groups highlighted in this article were formed to help members cope with the common problems that older people with mental illness face, and to maintain their residence in the least restrictive environment possible. Though many of the exclusionary criteria have a sound basis, they should point to possible barriers to mutual aid that the worker and the group members may have to address within the group.

One of the first tasks in the beginning phase of work is to develop a mutual agreement of the work the group will do together (Kurland &

Salmon, 1998; Northen & Kurland, 2001; Shulman, 1999). This task occurs during the initial stage of group development which has been described as a period of pre-affiliation (Garland, Jones, & Kolodny, 1965). In this stage of development it is not unusual for members to mistrust one another and the worker, be unable to see the connection among themselves, and to isolate. An approach-avoidance may occur towards the work and each other. When working with older persons with a mental illness, these member and group traits are likely to be magnified due to psychiatric symptoms and the diversity of life experiences brought to the group (e.g., early onset of mental illness as opposed to onset as an older person; varying functional levels and psychiatric symptomology).

In one of this author's groups there was a range of class, functional level, race, ethnicity, psychiatric diagnoses, ages (from 60-90). However most lived in varying levels of supported living, and all had problems in living secondary to mental illness and age. The initial mistrust and approach-avoidance centered on these composite differences. For example, higher functioning members would ignore lower functioning members, make disparaging comments about them, or would attempt to talk only to the worker. Rather than see these composite differences as reasons for exclusion from the group, the worker recognized them as obstacles to mutual aid. To remove this barrier, the worker helped members to see the mutual concerns and needs all members shared, pointed out how the group could help, and attempted to help members make connections with one another based on these shared concerns. Though the process took several months, members eventually saw the connections and made affectional ties. When the group was more developed members took on the responsibility of helping any new members see how the group could help with common concerns. For example, one new member began voicing concerns about all the "old mentally ill people" in the group. A veteran member from the same social background as the new member described how she felt the same way when she first came, but that she now found the group very helpful. She went on to describe the similarities between various members, how they had all helped one another, and invited the new member to give it a chance.

Authority and Intimacy Themes

Much has been written about stages of group development (e.g., Bennis & Shepard, 1956; Bion, 1961; Galinsky & Schopler, 1989; Garland, Jones, & Kolodny, 1965; Kelly & Berman-Rossi, 1999; Northen & Kurland, 2001; Schiller, 1997, 1995). Recent writings have begun to particularize group development theory to different settings and to different populations (e.g., Galinksy & Schopler; Kelly & Berman-Rossi; Schiller). It has become clear that not all groups develop in the same way, yet there are common themes that occur and issues that must be resolved as groups develop. These themes are the authority and intimacy themes (Bennis & Sheppard; Bion; Garland, Jones, & Kolodny). In order for the group as a whole to develop, these themes must be resolved enough for the group to get on with its identified work. We now know that exactly how and when groups address these issues depend on contextual and member factors as well as on worker skill. For groups for older adults living with chronic mental illness the emergence of these themes will be influenced by the members' histories, characteristics, and previous experiences.

The Authority Theme

One of the striking differences in groups for older persons with a mental illness can be the apparent lack of authority or power/control issues (Kelly, 1999). For those older persons who have spent many years in institutions, compliance, and dependency on staff were survival mechanisms. A "good patient" was a compliant patient. Others were socialized in an era when those in authority were to be respected, venerated, and listened to. In addition, vulnerable people are less likely to feel secure enough to challenge authority. As vulnerability is associated with old age and institutionalization (Kelly & Berman-Rossi, 1999; Berman-Rossi, 2001), it is not surprising that older adults with mental illness would have difficulty expressing any authority issues. However, workers must not be lulled into thinking that authority is not an issue. If one listens and looks closely, authority issues will be seen in non-traditional ways. If not dealt with, these can hinder the development of the group.

The most obvious way the authority theme will emerge in groups for mentally ill older people is through an exaggerated dependency upon the worker. Members may ask the worker to make all the decisions for them and tell them what to do. For example, Kelly (1999) describes a group interaction where something as small as asking a group member what she would like to drink during snack time provoked great anxiety. The member preferred to be told what to drink. Other examples include communication going through the worker, an expectation that the worker will decide upon and direct activities and discussion topics, or giving the worker the final say in discussions–even if wrong.

Worker: How is everyone this morning?

Members: Okay.

Worker: Last time we met we were talking about some of the problems everyone was having in their homes. Should we pick up on that discussion?

Members: Silently agree and shake their heads yes.

Worker: Tom, you were going to talk with your home provider about how you were tired of your food always being cold and not tasting good. How did that go?

Josh: Aw, that hateful woman just told me to stop complaining. She said she had lots of people to feed and hardly any money to do it on, so I should be grateful that I have good food to eat.

Members: (A few reported that they had complained in the past as well and were told similar things as Tom. The group members expressed hopelessness about being able to do anything to improve their situations, and they asked for the worker's help.)

Worker: Well it certainly must be rough to not like the food you are given to eat, but I am not sure what I can do to help. I wonder if the home providers are right. The State doesn't give much money to the home providers, and I am sure they are trying.

Josh: Yeah, they try, I guess.

Members: (All agree in resignation and sit in silence.)

Worker: Everyone sure is quiet.

Anne: Well it just seems hopeless so there is no point complaining. What else do you want us to talk about?

The unskillful practice example above illustrates how members allowed the worker to decide upon the topic, and when the worker sided with the powerful people in their lives, they withdrew and asked for the next topic rather than challenge his lack of empathy and understanding.

Later the worker revisited his poor practice and encouraged the members to challenge him. After many months of working with the group and actively encouraging their taking control of the group and challenging the worker, they began to do so. In another session several months later, the members began to complain about the route the van driver took everyday when bringing them to the center. The worker missed the authority challenge and sided with the van driver. The group erupted with anger at the worker for not listening to their concerns and after the worker apologized, the members came up with a workable solution on their own. The group had resolved the authority issue, but it took constant invitation over a long period of time.

Another way in which the authority theme may be different when working with older adults with a mental illness concerns differences between workers and group members. Composite differences between workers and group members can give rise to authority issues when working with any group. For example, in substance abuse groups it is not uncommon for members to challenge a worker without a substance abuse history. In parenting groups, a worker without children may be accused of not understanding how difficult raising children can be. These testing behaviors are often obvious and direct when working with younger groups. As described earlier, many older people were socialized to give authority figures their due respect, yet the authority (the worker) may be 50 or 60 years younger than the members. The normative testing that occurs in groups becomes complicated for older people with a mental illness as they need to test the worker to see if he or she understands, but testing of authority may be difficult due to socialization or for reasons of vulnerability. The testing may be very subtle or veiled, and the worker must listen very closely in order to encourage and engage the test. Questions about the age of the worker, remembering historical events (or not), or life experiences may be subtle tests to authority. In one group an African-American member raised in the Deep South during difficult racial times had been raised to call all white people "Mister" or "Miss" as a protective sign of respect. Even though first names were used in the group, she used the salutation when referring to white staff. Interestingly, this worker in authority was too young to be a "real Mister," so she always said "Mister Timmy!" This represented her ambivalence concerning age and authority. The first time Sandra said "Mr. Timmy" he commented on how he was too young to be "Mr. Tim" and she laughed and agreed. As the rest of the group began to laugh, the worker agreed with the group that he was rather "wet behind the ears" and asked the group to help "keep him straight." They agreed to help "educate" the worker, and then the worker asked Sandra if he could call her "Ms. Sandra." She laughed again, and agreed. This discussion opened up the authority theme and demonstrated that the worker was willing to engage directly with their feelings.

Intimacy

Intimacy in mutual aid groups is described by Berman-Rossi (1993) as a climate of trust where members increase self-revelation. Within such a climate of trust, members are able to discuss taboo subjects and take other risks. For many years it was common wisdom that groups could not move to the intimacy stage until the authority theme was dealt with. Schiller (1997, 1995) and Kelly and Berman-Rossi (1999) challenged the notion that authority precedes intimacy. For some vulnerable groups, safety and a sense of intimacy must develop *before* members are secure enough to openly deal with authority issues. This point is even more salient for many older adults with a mental illness. Though the research on social relationships for older people in general demonstrates, contrary to stereotypes and myths, that most older adults maintain meaningful social relationships (Cavanaugh, 1997; Johnson & Troll, 1994), older persons with a mental illness are often socially isolated and starved for connections with others. Hence they are less likely to risk losing any affectional ties.

Though the members in the author's groups did not initially engage the authority theme, it did not prevent the development of intimacy. As suggested in Schiller and later by Berman-Rossi and Kelly, a sense of security was required first. A growing climate of trust allowed members to begin taking risks and broaching taboo subjects. For example, the group members in the author's group discussed many taboo subjects including sexuality, aging, and death, and they sometimes were able to move into the topics with greater ease than the worker.

During one group session a member began to flirt with the worker, and he at first did not recognize what the behavior was. Only after other members began to tease the member and laugh at the worker's embarrassment was the worker able to broach the topic of sexuality. This opened up a discussion concerning how many of the members missed sexual expression and intimacy in their lives, and one member discussed her fears of contracting HIV from her boyfriend. The group worked with her overtime to try and reduce her high-risk sexual behavior. She was outwardly one of the most psychiatrically disabled members, yet she maintained a sexual relationship into her seventies.

Death was another taboo subject that members were able to openly discuss. In one poignant example, a member was discussing his rapidly failing health and his feelings that he would soon die. Another member asked him if he were ready to die. He said that he was ready, but that he was sad that his family, from whom he had been estranged for years, would not take notice that he was gone. The group began talking about how much they would miss him when he died. This lead to a discussion about death in general, and how much they meant to one another.

Potential Blocks to the Mutual Aid Process

All groups have the potential for mutual aid, yet many things can block the development. Shulman (1999) identifies these as: apparently divergent interests of group members, disruptive group roles and rules, and barriers to open communication. These potential blocks exist in groups for mentally ill older adults but, as with other group dynamics, these blocks may be qualitatively different. As described earlier, the multiplicity of life experiences secondary to race, class, gender, and psychiatric history accentuates diversity in older groups. This diversity of experience can make it more difficult for members to recognize their common interests, and presents many barriers to open communication.

Social norms, stereotypes, and taboos may also present barriers to open communication. For example, popular culture and socialization suggest that older people are not sexual beings. This may prevent some professionals from having discussions concerning sexuality with group members, yet mentally ill older adults have the need to openly discuss their sexual feelings. Taboos concerning death and illness may encourage younger workers to discourage open and frank discussions concerning death or cause workers to give false reassurances about health or long life.

A unique barrier to mutual aid for this group is paternalism. Older adults with mental illness are a vulnerable population, and this vulnerability may engender a paternalistic overprotectiveness in the worker. For example, Shulman (1999) identifies the dialectical process as one of the dynamics of mutual aid. In this process divergent ideas are expressed by members and in the process of discussing the divergent ideas, a new idea will emerge from the group. At times, the dialectical process will involve some group conflict. Working through group conflict, whether in the dialectical process or concerning a group issue, strengthens the group; however, protective feelings may cause the worker to preempt the conflict. For example, in one group the members were discussing medication compliance issues. Some of the members were saying that you had to take the medicine the psychiatrist prescribed no matter what. Others were saying that the doctors did not know anything and that they experimented on patients. This subgroup advocated just stopping the medicine if it did not agree with you. As the discussion became heated, the worker became concerned for the more vulnerable members and preempted the conflict by suggesting that taking medicine was very important and they must talk to their doctor if it did not agree with them. It would have been better for the worker to contain his protective feelings and help the members arrive at their own conclusion. Most likely, the members would have reached an agreement about the need to talk to doctors or other professionals about medication concerns.

CONCLUSION

Older adults with a mental illness are an extremely vulnerable group of people, and require extra environmental supports to face the numerous challenges they will encounter as they navigate the life transitions in the aging process. Group work can be such a powerful support. Unfortunately, most professionals would rather work with younger people (Litwin, 1994; Tan, Hawkins, & Ryan, 2001) as they are seen as more amenable to change, growth, and receiving benefit from services. In addition, persons with a chronic mental illness are thought to have little hope for psychological change and growth. As this article has demonstrated, both ideas are untrue. Changes may not be as dramatic as work with younger populations or with those groups coping with a life transition without the double jeopardy of a vulnerable life condition. However, older adults with a mental illness can and do change and grow, and receive great benefit from appropriate group work services.

Groups for this population function similarly to other groups, but the pace and way in which normative group issues and dynamics emerge will be influenced by the unique characteristics of the members. The worker must have group work knowledge and skill, and possess the ability to apply the knowledge and skills to a unique group of people. When this occurs, mutual aid can flourish and allow a vulnerable group to approach the end of their lives with dignity. There can be no more meaningful work than helping such vulnerable and marginalized people.

REFERENCES

Altholz, J. A. S. (1994). Group psychotherapy. In I. Burnside & M. Schmidt (Eds.), *Working with older adults: Group process and technique* (3rd ed.), pp. 214-224. Boston: Jones and Bartlett Publishers.

American Psychiatric Association (2000). *Diagnostic and statistical manual of mental disorder IV.* Washington: American Psychiatric Association Press.

Bennis, W., & Shepard, H. (1956). A theory of group development. *Human Relations, 9, 415-437.*

Berman-Rossi, T. (2001). Older persons in need of long-term care. In A. Gitterman (Ed.), *Handbook of social work practice with vulnerable and resilient populations* (2nd ed.), pp. 715-768. New York: Columbia University Press.

Berman-Rossi, T. (1990). Group work and older persons. In A. Monk (Ed.), *Handbook of gerontological services* (2nd ed.), pp. 141-167. New York: Columbia University Press.

Berman-Rossi, T. (1993). The tasks and skills of the social worker across stages of group development. *Social Work with Groups, 16*(1/2), 69-81.

Berman-Rossi, T., & Cohen, M. B. (1989). Group decision making working with homeless mentally ill women. *Social Work with Groups, 11*(4), 63-78.

Bion, W. R. (1959). *Experiences in groups.* New York: Ballantine Books.

Blankenship, L. M., Molinari, V., & Kunik, M. (1996). The effect of a life review group on the reminiscence functions of geropsychiatric inpatients. *Clinical Gerontologist, 16*(4), 3-18.

Burnside, I., & Schmidt, M. G. (1994). Demographic and psychosocial aspects of aging. In I. Burnside, & M. Schmidt (Eds.), *Working with older adults: Group process and technique* (3rd ed.), pp. 8-23. Boston: Jones and Bartlett Publishers.

Cavanaugh, J. C. (1997). *Adult development and aging* (3rd ed.). Pacific Grove, CA: Brooks/Cole Publishing Company.

Garland, J., Jones, H., & Kolodny, R. (1965). A model for stages of development I social work groups. In S. Bernstein (Ed.), *Explorations in group work: Essays in theory and practice,* pp. 12-53. Boston: Boston University School of Social Work.

Gitterman, A. (1994). Developing a new group service. In A. Gitterman & L. Shulman (Eds.), *Mutual aid groups, vulnerable populations, and the life cycle* (2nd ed.), pp. 59-77. New York: Columbia University Press.

Gray, C. A., & Geron, S. M. (1995). The other sorrow of divorce: The effects on grandparents when their adult children divorce. *Journal of Gerontological Social Work, 23*(3/4), 139-159.

Husaini, B. A., Moore, S. T., & Cain, V. A. (1994). Psychiatric symptoms and help-seeking behavior among the elderly: An analysis of racial and gender differences. *Journal of Gerontological Social Work, 21*(3/4), 177-195.

Johnson, C. L., & Troll, L. E. (1994). Constraints and facilitators to friendships in late life. *The Gerontologist, 34*(1), 79-87.

Kelly, T. B. (1999). Mutual aid groups with mentally ill older adults. *Social Work with Groups, 21*(4), 63-80.

Kelly, T. B., & Berman-Rossi, T. (1999). Advancing stages of group development theory: The case of institutionalized older persons. *Social Work with Groups,* 22(2/3), 119-138.

Kennedy, G. J. (2000). *Geriatric mental health care.* New York: Guilford Press.

Kurland, R. (1978). Planning: The neglected component of group development. *Social Work with Groups, 1*(2), 173-178.

Kurland, R., & Salmon, R. (1998). *Teaching a methods course in social work with groups.* Alexandria, VA: Council on Social Work Education.

Lagana, L., & Shanks, S. (2002). Mutual biases underlying the problematic relationship between older adults and mental health providers: Any solution in sight? *International Journal of Aging & Human Development, 55*(3), 271- 295.

Lesser, J., Lazarus, L. W., Frankel, R., & Havasy, S. (1981). Reminiscence group therapy with psychotic geriatric inpatients. *The Gerontologist, 21*(3), 291-296.

Litwin, H. (1994). The professional standing of work with elderly persons among social work trainees. *British Journal of Social Work, 24*(1), 53-69.

Lowy, L. (1985). *Social work with the aging: The challenge and promise of the later years* (2nd ed.). Prospect Heights, IL: Waveland Press, Inc.

Lowy, L. (1983). Social group work with vulnerable older persons: A theoretical perspective. In S. Saul (Ed.), *Group work with the frail elderly,* pp. 21-32. New York: The Haworth Press, Inc.

Meeks, S., & Hammond, C. T. (2001). Social network characteristics among older outpatients with a long-term mental illness. *Journal of Mental Health and Aging, 7*(4), 445-464.

Northen, H., & Kurland, R. (2001). *Social work with groups* (3rd ed.). New York: Columbia University Press.

Padgett, D. K., Burns, B. J., & Grau, L. A. (1988). Risk factors and resilience. In B. L. Levin, A. K. Blanch, & A. Jennings (Eds.), *Women's mental health services* pp. 390-413. Thousand Oaks, CA: Sage.

Raschko, R. (1991) Spokane Community Mental Health Center elderly services. In E. Light & B. D. Lebowitz (Eds.), *The elderly with chronic mental illness,* pp. 232-244. New York: Springer Publishing Company.

Rose, M. K., Soares, H. H., & Joseph, C. (1993). Frail elderly clients with personality disorders: A challenge for social work. *Journal of Gerontological Social Work, 19*(3/4), 153-165.

Schiller, L. Y. (1997). Rethinking stages of group development in women's groups: Implications for practice. *Social Work with Groups, 20*(3), 3-19.

Schiller, L. Y. (1995). Stages of development in women's groups: A relational model. In R. Kurland & R. Salmon (Eds.), *Group work practice in a troubled society: Problems and opportunities,* pp. 117-138. New York: The Haworth Press, Inc.

Shulman, L. (1999). *The skills of helping individuals, families, groups, and communities.* Itasca, IL: F. E. Peacock Publishers, Inc.

Stoller, E. P., & Gibson, R. C. (2000). *Worlds of difference: Inequality in the aging experience.* Thousand Oaks, CA: Pine Forge Press.

Tan, P. P., Hawkins, M. P., & Ryan, E. (2001). Baccalaureate social work student attitudes toward older adults. *Journal of Baccalaureate Social Work, 6*(2), 45-55.

Toseland, R. W. (1995). *Group work with the elderly.* New York: Springer Publishing Company.

Zarit, S. H., & Zarit, J. M. (1998). *Mental disorders in older adults: Fundamentals of assessment and treatment.* New York: Guilford.

The Relationship
Between Caregiver Support Groups
and the Marker Framework of Caregiving

Helene Ebenstein, MSW

SUMMARY. This article explores the relationship between caregiver support groups and the marker framework of family caregiving. Group workers knowledgeable about the various stages or markers in the career of a caregiver and the issues which precipitate moving to a new marker are better able to assist the group and its members. The five markers most relevant to caregiver support groups are: (1) self-definition as a caregiver, (2) performing personal care, (3) seeking assistance and formal service use, (4) consideration of nursing home placement, and (5) termination of the caregiving role. The marker framework is a valuable tool to aid group workers in effectively marketing groups, selecting members and enhancing support of the group. *[Article copies available for a fee from The Haworth Document Delivery Service: 1-800-HAWORTH. E-mail address: <docdelivery@haworthpress.com> Website: <http://www. HaworthPress.com> © 2004 by The Haworth Press, Inc. All rights reserved.]*

KEYWORDS. Caregiver career, caregiver support groups, family caregiving, group work, marker framework of caregiving

---

[Haworth co-indexing entry note]: "The Relationship Between Caregiver Support Groups and the Marker Framework of Caregiving." Ebenstein, Helene. Co-published simultaneously in *Journal of Gerontological Social Work* (The Haworth Social Work Practice Press, an imprint of The Haworth Press, Inc.) Vol. 44, No. 1/2, 2004, pp. 127-149; and: *Group Work and Aging: Issues in Practice, Research, and Education* (ed: Robert Salmon, and Roberta Graziano) The Haworth Social Work Practice Press, an imprint of The Haworth Press, Inc., 2004, pp. 127-149. Single or multiple copies of this article are available for a fee from The Haworth Document Delivery Service [1-800-HAWORTH, 9:00 a.m. - 5:00 p.m. (EST). E-mail address: docdelivery@ haworthpress.com].

INTRODUCTION

Just as support groups go through stages, family caregivers pass through stages of caregiving. (The stages of group development are used extensively in both the theory and practice of group work. For examples, see Garland, Jones, & Kolodny, 1973; Kelly & Berman-Rossi, 1999; Junn-Krebs, 2003; Kurland & Salmon, 1998; Northen & Kurland, 2001; Schiller, 1995; Toseland, 1995). Although there is wide diversity among caregivers, uniform events often mark the shift from one stage to the next. For group members caring for a relative with a chronic debilitating illness, there is little likelihood that recovery will end caregiving responsibilities. In most cases, caregivers foresee a future of increasing responsibility and the decline of the relative ending with death. Since most caregiver support groups have members in various stages of their caregiving "career," group leaders familiar with the caregiving trajectory can help support group members navigate the difficult transitions they face. Understanding which events lead to a new stage and the feelings that result enable a worker to facilitate more effectively.

The myth that family members in the United States do not take responsibility for caring for a relative has been firmly debunked in survey after survey. A 1997 survey estimated that there were 22.4 million caregivers in the United States. An astonishing one in four households contained a family caregiver. The survey predicted that by the year 2007 the number of caregiving households for people aged 50 and over could reach 39 million (National Alliance for Caregiving/AARP, 1997). About two-thirds of older people living in the community and needing long-term care depend on family and friends. Only 8% depend entirely on paid help (Liu, Manton, & Aragon, 2000). The estimated value of care provided by family caregivers is staggering. Arno et al. estimated it at $196 billion in 1997 (Arno, Levine, & Memmott, 1999). The number of caregivers and the demands on them continue to grow rapidly as older people live longer with chronic illnesses, are discharged earlier from hospitals and rely more on outpatient care (Houts, Nezu, Nezu, & Bucher, 1996).

Although caregivers often talk of the satisfactions and rewards of caregiving, there are also many negative consequences. Caregivers report higher levels of stress, burden and depression (Fredman & Daly, 1998; The Henry J. Kaiser Family Foundation, 2002) as well as physical problems associated with caregiving (Schulz, O'Brien, Bookwala, & Fleissner, 1995) which may even lead to death (Schulz & Beach, 1999).

The financial cost is also high. In addition to out-of-pocket expenses, a 1996 survey found that many caregivers made adjustments in their work schedule, worked fewer hours, retired early or quit the work force (Feder, Komisar, & Niefeld, 2000).

When caregivers are asked how health care workers can help, they mention information, education, respite care and emotional support as their highest priorities (Levine, 1999). A small but significant number consider caregiver support groups. How can we help to make their experience in a caregiver support group as positive and valuable as possible? So much is expected of family caregivers and they expect so little in return. As Carol Levine (1999) writes, "No one advocates on my husband's behalf except me: No one advocates on my behalf, not even me." (p. 1588). When they consider a support group, caregivers have the right to expect a group worker sensitive to the caregiving experience, familiar with the stresses as well as the rewards, and knowledgeable about resources. Awareness of caregiving markers and their significance will help workers meet those expectations.

This paper will describe the "marker framework" of caregiving (Montgomery & Kosloski, 2001) and highlight the five markers which are most relevant to support groups for caregivers of the chronically ill elderly:

1. Self-definition as a Caregiver,
2. Performing Personal Care,
3. Seeking Assistance and Formal Service Use,
4. Consideration of Nursing Home Placement, and
5. Termination of the Caregiving Role.

The intent of this discussion is to heighten the awareness of group workers to the importance of these markers and to help prepare them for the difficulties which group members may be experiencing at these times. Examples of group process from the caregiver support group facilitated by the author will illustrate how one group deals with these transitions and attempts to assist members in handling them.

CAREGIVER SUPPORT GROUPS

Do caregivers actually benefit from membership in a support group? Surprisingly, there is disagreement on this question. Benefits can be defined as decreased depression or burden, increased satisfaction, increased use of other formal services and/or delay in institutionalization. Results of research seeking to determine if caregiver stress is lowered or caregiver satisfaction is raised have been mixed (Monahan, 1994). Researchers also explore the relationship between support groups and the use of other formal services such as adult day care (Bass, McCarthy, Eckert, & Bichler, 1994). One study showed that problem-focused coping strategies were more effective in reducing depression than emotion-focused strategies (Batt-Leiba, Hills, Johnson, & Bloch, 1998). Some studies compare the effectiveness of support groups to more structured educational programs. Others suggest that a combination is most beneficial to family caregivers (Cummings, 1996). Perhaps there is no "one size fits all" approach. Clearly, some people seek out support groups and remain in them during their years of caregiving. They must be getting something positive from group membership. The Alzheimer's Association in the New York City area alone sponsors more than 100 caregiver support groups. Since many caregivers are unable to attend support groups due to their caregiving responsibilities, groups are increasingly offered over the telephone and even online (Kelly, 1997).

Caregivers who are asked what they get out of support groups mention being with people having similar experiences, receiving emotional support, problem resolution, getting information on community supports, and learning caregiving skills (Kaye & Applegate, 1993). This list challenges the group worker to be knowledgeable about legal issues, community resources, entitlements, the difficulty of combining formal and informal services, techniques of dealing with difficult behaviors, and home care management. Familiarity with emotional and social issues such as family conflict over caregiving, coping with loss, grief, and issues of self-esteem are essential as well as a firm grounding in group dynamics. Important, too, is helping members balance the difficult realities of caregiving with hope, pride in accomplishment, and humor (Kaye & Applegate, 1993; Monahan, 1994). There is also discussion of whether it is best to offer separate groups, depending on caregiver relationship, culture, or illness, or mix all caregivers together in one group. Monahan states that more positive outcomes are associated with groups targeted to specific audiences (Monahan, 1994). One underlying theme is the special burden carried by caregivers of people with dementia. More than dealing with a relative's physical needs, caregivers suffer most because of unusual, unpredictable, and sometimes dangerous behaviors. The agony of watching a family member die a little more each day is especially devastating (Prigerson, 2003; Sanders & Corley, 2003). As one group member put it, "There is a reason they call Alzheimer's Disease the long goodbye." Support groups provide a resource that can be relied on over an often very long career of caregiving (McCallion & Toseland, 1995).

MARKER FRAMEWORK OF CAREGIVING

The marker framework of caregiving developed by Montgomery and Kosloski recognizes the diversity of caregiver experiences but also the patterns of the experience (Montgomery & Kosloski, 2001). The marker framework is useful in understanding how to meet the needs of different caregivers and market support services to caregivers when they are most receptive to the services. It has been applied to explain and address caregiver reluctance to take advantage of community services offered. Programs designed to give caregivers the services they say they need, including support groups, are consistently underused. The marker framework is useful to support group workers in recruiting new members and in facilitating the group meetings. The framework enriches understanding of the caregiver experience and attitudes affecting the decision to join and participate in a support group. Although there are a total of seven markers in the framework, this paper will highlight the five markers most relevant to support groups.

The illustrative examples are based on the author's experiences as a group worker in a support group for adult children caring for a family member with dementia. The group, sponsored by the Alzheimer's Association, has been meeting for four years and the author has led the group for the past three. The group meets in a large urban hospital every other week in the evenings. Group composition changes over time as family members die or caregivers leave the group and new caregivers join. Current members range in age from 33 to 67 and are evenly divided between men and women. All parents are in the middle to late stages of their illness. Three members live with their parents. The other parents are at home with home care, in an assisted living facility, or in a nursing home.

Self-Definition as a Caregiver

At what point does a family member become a caregiver? For some the transition is dramatic. Serious injury in an automobile accident or paralysis due to a stroke thrusts a family member into the unwanted career of family caregiver (Levine,1999). For most, though, the path to caregiving is gradual. Concern for a forgetful spouse or parent may evolve over time into increasing supervision and responsibility. Family members are not eager to see themselves as caregivers, preferring to view their role as, for example, a helpful wife or simply doing what any son would do (Dobrof, Zodikoff, Ebenstein, & Phillips, 2002). For spouses, in particular, the process is devastating. Cummings describes how "spousal caregivers are faced with the continual challenge of read-justing their understanding of their relationship with their partner and their participation in that relationship" (Cummings,1996). "Taking on the role of caregiver involves taking on something new, but is also about loss of what was–or was to be" (Dobrof & Ebenstein, 2003-2004).

Both the difficulty in determining at what point family members "drift" into the role of caregiver and the reluctance to see themselves in this role is important for support group workers to note on behalf of both the individual and the group. An AARP study indicates that early self-identification benefits the caregiver, leading to more activities helpful in managing responsibilities, learning more about caregiving, or asking for help before a crisis (Kutner, 2001). On the other hand, unless pro-spective group members see themselves as caregivers, they will not be able to identify with other group members in a mutually supportive way. It is also unlikely that they will stay in the group for very long. This might be relevant when, for example, a prospective group member has just learned of a family member's diagnosis and rushes to join a support group to learn more about the illness. Since the public is becoming more aware of illnesses such as Alzheimer's Disease and diagnoses are made earlier, this scenario will occur more frequently (Feinberg & Ellano, 2000). Pressure from family, friends or health care workers may also prompt a premature contact about joining a support group.

There is no simple method of gauging readiness to join a support group based on the length of time since diagnosis or the stage of the dis-ease. Caregivers move from marker to marker at differing paces and don't necessarily follow the marker order suggested by Montgomery and Kosloski. However, the research of Bass et al. indicated that sup-port groups tend to be used by caregivers later in the disease process (Bass et al., 1994). When interviewing prospective group members, support group workers knowledgeable about the difficulty of self-defi-nition will be better able to explore this issue, encourage self-identifica-tion and help insure that those joining the group are ready to do so. For those who do not identify as caregivers, it might be better to suggest first attending educational workshops and learning more about caregiving before joining a group. This strategy is appropriate if, in the worker's view, a prospective group member would have difficulty connecting with other group members at this stage. Without the all-in-the-same-boat communal feeling, the power of the group will be compromised (Shulman, 1999, pp. 306-307).

The following illustrative example took place in the support group facilitated by the author.

Maryanne's father was recently diagnosed with Alzheimer's Disease. She contacted the group worker who arranged for an interview. During the interview the group worker explored with Maryanne her feelings about being in a group with people caring for parents in various stages of Alzheimer's Disease including the later stages. The group worker suspected that Maryanne's father was actually farther along in the disease process than she was acknowledging. Whether Maryanne saw herself as a caregiver, a more basic issue, was not adequately explored.

At the first support group meeting Maryanne attended, the following interchange took place towards the end of the session:

Maryanne: I don't know if I belong in this group. Everyone else has a parent who is in really bad shape and you are all doing so much to help them. My father is in the very early stages. He is actually sweeter than he's ever been. All I do is visit him.

Robert: But you said that your father almost never leaves his room anymore and you keep trying to get him to go for walks and things.

Nora: And your mother doesn't accept that anything is wrong with your father and the two of you keep fighting over this.

Maryanne: I know, but my father is really doing well now. He can take care of himself.

Group worker: Maryanne, what was it like for you hearing about parents who are in worse shape than your father?

Maryanne: It's hard to hear but one of the reasons I came to the group is to prepare myself for down the road.

In this example, Maryanne does not see herself in the same boat as the other group members. Group members offer a differing view based on what Maryanne has told them. Although they point out the ways in which she is a caregiver, Maryanne is not convinced. The worker continues to focus on the possibility that Maryanne is afraid to think about the future deterioration in her father's condition. Although this is probably a factor, the overriding issue is Maryanne's view that she is not a caregiver and, therefore, does not belong in a caregiver support group.

Maryanne came to the next two meetings and then decided that she did not need a support group at this time. Nearly one year later she rejoined the support group. Maryanne became an active, committed group member when her father's condition reached the point that she saw herself as his caregiver. That occurred when her father needed help with personal care.

Performing Personal Care

This stage is reached when the caregiver begins helping with tasks such as bathing, dressing, or toileting. It is often a turning point for caregivers in several ways. Reaching this stage highlights the changing relationship between caregiver and care recipient, may trigger consider- ation of the use of formal service or placement and often results in conflicts among family members. The gradual assumption of other care- giving tasks, such as banking, shopping and meal preparation can still be viewed by family members as "just lending a hand" or "doing what any wife would do." This view does not change the basic relationship that had previously existed between the caregiver and the care recipient. This is especially true for spouses who might have had many of these responsibilities before the decline of their partner. Once there is a need for help with personal care, however, the change in the dynamics of the relationship becomes clearer. The need to assist with personal care may be the point that a caregiver first self-identifies. It may also be the time that a caregiver considers formal service use or nursing home placement. It is possible, therefore, that a caregiver may be reaching several stages of caregiving simultaneously. Clearly, reaching this point in the caregiving career is extremely traumatic. Caregivers are juggling a host of responsibilities as well as dealing with feelings such as grief, loss, disappointment, and anger. Disagreements among family members often come to the fore around decisions regarding how to care for a family member, who will provide the care and the cost of care. These issues stress the family system even when it usually functions well.

The difficulties may be compounded by the reactions of the care recipient, especially when dementia is involved. Caregivers struggle when their attempts, for example, to shower a family member result in physical resistance, shouting, and crying. They wonder how their good intentions can lead to such painful interactions and distress for all. Nora, a group member, describes how she is often in tears after trying to bathe her mother. Other group members shake their heads in recognition and sympathy.

Despite these problems, it is also important to keep in mind the rewards of caregiving often noted by caregivers and to help group members express feelings of satisfaction, accomplishment, and honor. Kaye and Applegate (1993) noted that support groups can be depressing and demoralizing if only the pain and suffering are dealt with at meetings. Although not true for every caregiver, many feel proud of what they are doing and honored that they can be of help to a loved one. Group members are "amazed" at what they have been able to handle and "grateful" that they are there for a parent who has given them so much. These feelings help to temper the stresses and revitalize the caregiver. Encouraging humor is also essential. Barry told the group he would never be able to attend the meetings if there wasn't also a "chance to have a good laugh."

Issues raised at this stage are especially suitable for caregiver support groups. Group members will find they are not alone in feeling angry with other family members or overwhelmed by the deterioration of a once-competent family member. The group can help each other through mutual support, sharing information and experiences, discussing the pros and cons of various decision options, and individual problem solving (Steinberg, 1997). Group workers familiar with family dynamics and grief work, strategies for dealing with difficult behaviors, use of social supports, and community resources, will be most effective.

The following interchange from the Adult Children's Group is illustrative:

Maryanne, who was mentioned above, returned to the group after her father's condition deteriorated. She was the first to speak at one group meeting.

Maryanne: Last week was very rough. I visited my father in his room and as soon as I walked in there was a horrible smell. I found him with no clothes on, sitting in his own feces, watching television. My father was the most private, proud man. He didn't even seem embarrassed or realize that anything was wrong. To think that I used to be so afraid of him and now he is helpless.

Nora: This disease is so terrible. I'm watching my mother, my best friend, go through changes like that, too, and there is nothing that anyone can do to stop it (Nora begins to cry). I feel so helpless.

Betty: (Reaches over to touch Nora's shoulder) Maryanne, is your father taking Aricept?

Group worker: Betty, let's stay with these feelings for a while. How is it for you to see changes in your mother?

Betty: Very, very painful. We were always very close. My mother was the kindest, most dignified person I know but now she does things that she would be mortified doing. That hurts me so. (Betty has tears in her eyes) But despite everything, I thank God that I'm around to help her get good care (Nora nods in agreement).

Maryanne: You know what's especially hard for me. My father and I were never close. He was a cold disciplinarian. It's strange. I feel closer to him now than I ever did. But things with my mother are going downhill. My mother refuses to see that anything is really wrong. She hardly sees my father and doesn't take care of him. And I think she doesn't want to spend money on hiring someone. Am I crazy to think that I should stop working and spend my time taking care of him?

Betty: That's a big decision. I think that you have to think this out carefully before you do something like that.

Ed: Do you really want to or do you feel that you should do it?

Maryanne: Maybe I'm just trying to show my mother how lousy she is acting. I guess that's not a realistic plan.

Group worker: Maryanne, you are dealing with a lot right now. Maybe the group can help you sort out some of the options.

　　The group then talked with Maryanne about strategies for approaching her mother, various ways to care for her father, and the worker supplemented the discussion with information on home care and residential resources. Several months after this interchange, Maryanne convinced her mother to move her father to an assisted living facility that she learned of in the group.

In this interaction, group members supported each other in expressing their pain and also touched on the rewards of caregiving. The group worker led Betty away from the concrete and asked her to react to the feelings expressed by others. When Maryanne raised the possibility of providing hands-on care for her father, the reaction of two group members helped her reconsider. The worker then asked the group to work on helping Maryanne with a problem that seemed overwhelming.

Seeking Assistance and Formal Service Use

Researchers consistently find that caregivers, even those providing intensive home care, make little use of community services (Montgomery & Borgatta, 1989). Most families provide care for an ill relative for many years before even considering formal services such as home care, adult day programs, home delivered meals (Gottlieb & Johnson, 2000) There are many reasons for this reluctance. Caregivers feel that they can and should be able to handle everything without assistance, the family is skeptical of the quality of care, and the caregiver fears handing over control to outsiders (Collins et al., 1991). Seeking assistance is also an acknowledgement that the caregiving situation has progressed to another stage in the relative's deterioration. To add to the dilemma, care recipients often adamantly refuse. In a 1998 survey of caregivers, 37% said that the care recipient did not want strangers in their home (The Henry J. Kaiser Family Foundation, 2002). Although Montgomery and Kosloski (2001) include joining a support group or attending educational programs in this marker, the author's experience has been that it is the use of in-home care or adult day programs that is most significant in defining this stage of the caregiving career. There is also evidence that differences in seeking assistance and accepting formal care may be attributed to the relationship and gender of the caregiver.

For many caregivers the decision to accept formal service is painful and made during a crisis when there is no other choice. Caregivers see respite care as "an end-of-the-road service to be used when they are on the verge of breaking down" (Brody, Saperstein, & Lawton, 1989, p. 69). The worker's awareness of the symbolic meanings attached to formal service use is important in many group work interactions. Helping group members discuss the meanings they associate with formal service will bring the feelings of shame, guilt, anger, and failure out in the open, facilitating the all-in-the-same-boat phenomenon. Imagine the relief of group members who realize that others are struggling with the same feelings regardless of where they stand on the issue. Encouraging nonjudgmental interactions between those group members already using outside help and those who are not benefits all members, leading to mutual support and empathy. The group leader's sensitivity in handling these discussions can help members feel supported by each other. Asking group members who are using formal services how they handled the objections of the care recipient and/or other family members critical of their decision, can generate an exchange of ideas and tips. This sharing of data assists members considering formal service who anticipate negative reactions. Rehearsing or role playing is useful in preparing a group member for a difficult conversation with a family member. Simply discussing the issue helps to normalize its use, removing it from the unspoken or taboo. The group worker's skill and knowledge can also help the group support a desperate caregiver who cannot bear to enter this new stage of caregiving.

Familiarity with community resources and how they are accessed is also essential here. The worker is responsible for being up-to-date, educating group members about possible services and their costs and entitlements, and providing contact information. Another important responsibility is explaining the range of care available. Caregivers sometimes have the misconception that accepting formal care means, for example, accepting 24-hour live-in care. By clarifying the possibility of beginning slowly and increasing services in time, an overwhelmed caregiver may begin to see a way out. Often group members have much of the knowledge outlined above and will take responsibility for educating the others. But the worker must be ready to correct misinformation or provide further details, as needed.

The following occurred in the Adult Children's Group:

Barry's mother, who lived alone 100 miles away, was diagnosed with dementia three years ago. Barry saw her every weekend and helped with shopping and bill paying. A neighbor came in for a few hours three times a week to help his mother with meals and laundry but she had recently told Barry that she would soon be moving away. In previous meetings, Barry talked about his mother's decline with deep concern but was resistant to gentle suggestions by group members that she might need more care at home. The group worker had tried to help the group explore with Barry what a change in home care arrangements might signify. Barry had missed the previous meeting so when he arrived at the next one, the group worker asked:

Group worker: Barry, I know that you weren't able to attend the last meeting because of a problem with your mother. How are things going there?

Barry: I'm a wreck and I'm so angry at people who keep interfering when they have no business getting involved.

Ed: What happened?

Barry: It's been a nightmare. A few weeks ago I got a call from a neighbor telling me that my mother was wandering around the street at night and fell. She didn't fall because she was wandering! She went out for a walk and had a mild heart attack. She was all right though. Then a few days later I got a call from the police. They had some nerve. The officer told me that my mother was wandering and not dressed appropriately and they heard from neighbors that this had happened before. He said that if I didn't do something about it, he would. Can you believe that? I'm furious with him and the neighbors.

Nora: Where is your mother now?

Barry: I took off from work and I've been staying with her in her house. I just came home today.

Nora: Did you get someone to stay with your mother?

Barry: No. My mother doesn't want any strangers in the house. She likes the neighbor who comes a few times a week but the neighbor can't give her any more time. I don't know what to do. I think she would be happier in an assisted living place because she is sociable but she wants to stay in her home. Also, I have no idea who I could get to stay with her. Maybe I can start visiting assisted living places.

Susan: But Barry, you can't leave your mother alone while you're checking them out.

Barry: I think she'll be OK.

(There is silence.)

Group worker: What do people think?

(There is silence.)

Group worker: I wonder what people are saying by their silence.

Ed: I think your mother needs someone living with her now.

Barry: But I can't stay any longer. I have to go back to work.

Robert: I had to make a hard decision with my mother when I put her in the assisted living facility. I'll probably feel guilty about that for the rest of my life. But I couldn't move her in with me and I couldn't stay home and care for her. Sometimes you just have to do what you don't want to do. Your mother has a home she loves. Why not try to get someone to stay with her there?

Barry: I would try if I knew how to find someone.

Group worker: I have some information on places that you can call for a live-in worker. If you'd like, I'll call you first thing tomorrow morning.

Barry: Thanks. I'd appreciate that.

One week later, using a source provided by another group member, Barry located a home attendant who moved into his mother's home. After a rocky few weeks, she and Barry's mother adjusted well and the attendant is still there eight months later.

This interchange demonstrates the power of the group in a variety of ways. Barry used the group as a sounding board, presenting his view of the situation. Although group members were first reluctant to disagree, with the assistance of the group worker, a differing view was expressed. This exchange of views is essential to the mutual aid process. Robert, who had also faced a difficult decision, empathically shared his feelings about the experience. The group members cared enough about Barry to, in effect, demand very gently that he take the next step at the time that he was feeling overwhelmed and helpless (Shulman, 1999, pp. 308- 309). Finally, the group worker offered to provide concrete information to help Barry get the service he needed. In the end, it was another group member who helped him locate a home attendant.

Consideration of Nursing Home Placement

This marker is reached when a caregiver seriously considers placing a family member in a nursing home as an alternative to whatever arrangement currently exists. Caregivers vary widely in when, if ever, they reach this marker. For some, the difficulty of managing disruptive behaviors or the realization that at least some assistance with personal care is needed, precipitates the possibility of nursing home placement. Other caregivers are determined that no matter what state a family member is in, nursing home placement will not be considered. There are also many caregivers who have made promises to never place a relative in a nursing home. There is no guarantee, however, that the caregiver is at peace with that promise. As with other markers, this one is usually reached when there is a crisis, a sharp decline in the family member's condition or some event which upsets the existing care plan.

Group workers who understand the inevitability of this marker and its significance will be prepared when it arises in the group. Whether or not other members have raised the issue, it is often a flash point for all. Some members may be critical of anyone even considering this move. Members may also feel threatened and worried that they, too, may eventually face a similar situation. A member who has already placed a care recipient in a nursing home may feel criticized or attacked. Guilt is an underlying current.

The importance of encouraging discussion of this taboo topic cannot be overstated. Group members must address the "elephant in the room" in an open, nonthreatening way. The group worker's skill and knowledge are essential here. Sometimes educating members to a full range of options can reduce the pressure on caregivers. Many are unaware that in-home care is a possible alternative. Assisted living arrangements may be another option which group members may have heard about but only vaguely understand. Knowledge of entitlement programs such as Medicaid and delivered meal programs is also important. Group workers are responsible for insuring that various viewpoints are expressed, and any members who have made a promise to never consider nursing home placement have the opportunity to talk about that promise that may have become an unbearable burden. Finally, the group worker's awareness of his/her own point of view on this emotional issue and the possibility of countertransference are important to bear in mind.

Consideration of nursing home placement was discussed in the following interchange from the Adult Children's Caregiver Support Group.

Caroline, a 33-year-old caregiver, was unusually quiet and looked preoccupied. Midway through the session, the group worker turned to Caroline.

Group worker: Caroline, you seem to be somewhere else tonight.

Caroline: A lot has happened since the last time I was here. Just about everything went wrong. My mother totally flipped out. She started crying and shaking and throwing things. I called 911 and she's been in the hospital ever since. I decided I can't handle things at home any longer. If I'm going to keep my sanity I think I have to place her in a nursing home. I want to have a relationship, have a family and my life has been on hold for three years. (Caroline is in tears)

Ed: Is there anything wrong with her physically?

Susan: What if she doesn't want to go?

Group worker: Let's stay with how Caroline is feeling about this.

Caroline: I feel terrible and guilty but I can't continue to care for her at home, work full time, and have any kind of life for myself. It will be the hardest thing I've ever done.

Albert: I could never do it. I'd be worried about my mother all the time even though living with her drives me so crazy. Besides, I promised my mother that I would never do that.

Kara: My mother made me promise never to put her in a nursing home but I cared for her for a long time and it got to be too much. My whole family was affected. In the end I decided I had to put her in a nursing home. And you know who was all upset about it? The family members who never did anything. They all had something to say then. Albert, sometimes you have to save yourself. I would never, ever want my children to go through what we are going through. The person I'm most worried about is you, not your mother.

In this interchange, the group worker, by turning to Caroline, encouraged her to raise a taboo topic. Two other members immediately went to the concrete issues, possibly to avoid staying on this uncomfortable subject. The group worker firmly kept the focus on the feelings surrounding this topic. This allowed Caroline to express her feelings and other members to share their views. The group was able to express differing views in a supportive way. It is possible that Albert may reconsider his decision to never even consider placement. As of this writing, Caroline's mother remains at home. The group supported her efforts to request additional hours of home care from Medicaid which relieved some of the pressure on her.

Termination of Caregiving Role

Eventually the responsibility of caregiving comes to an end. The family member being cared for may die or recover or the caregiver may give up the responsibility of caregiving. It is important to be aware that placement in a nursing home or other institution does not end the caregiving role. In almost all instances, the caregiver continues to oversee the care of the family member, visit, and provide care.

The most common reason for the termination of the caregiving role for the chronically ill elderly is death. Caregivers struggle with a wide range of emotions and feelings in dealing with the death of the family member–grief, relief, guilt, and a feeling of emptiness and loss of purpose are just a few (Shenk, 2001). Group workers have a twofold responsibility to support group members regarding the termination of the caregiving role–to help prepare members to deal with the eventual termination and to support those members who are dealing with the loss of their caregiving role.

These responsibilities coincide when a group member experiences the death of the person for whom they are caring. The worker focuses on the member who suffered the loss but is also mindful of the effect that this event has on all group members. Encouraging the group member to continue coming to the group helps ease the transition from the caregiving role to its termination. Although the caregiver's life and routine are changing dramatically, the routine of attending the group and getting support from trusted members can comfort. Group members who have had this experience state that group meetings are the only time they feel comfortable expressing the full range of emotions raised by the death of the care recipient, especially those that might upset friends or other family members. Perhaps these meetings are the only outlet for expressing relief, anger at the dead family member, and/or fear of the future without the anchor of caregiving. The worker's role here is to encourage the expression of the gamut of emotions, to help normalize them, and to support adjusting to the end of the caregiving role. Assisting members in reviewing their accomplishments throughout the years in the face of many problems is important. Members' advice to each other to "Give yourself credit, not guilt" is healing.

Other group members are usually profoundly affected by the event. The member's loss is likely to engender expressions of sympathy, concern, and support. One of the benefits of a mutual aid group is the chance for members to help each other and this opportunity is positive and satisfying. There are other opportunities, however, which the group worker may need to help the group take advantage of. This includes the expression of emotions or feelings that may not be seen as so supportive or generous but must still be brought into the open. Envy that a member's ordeal is over while yours continues is one possibility. Criticism of a member's reaction to the death or blame for the death are other possibilities. There is also the chance to see a group member survive and adjust to the end of the caregiving role. Those who are extremely anxious about the inevitable death of a family member will have a model to observe and learn from. If the transition is very complicated, the group can also learn from that. The group worker's job is complex and requires balancing the needs of all members.

Other opportunities may arise which allow the group to deal with the eventual death of a family member in less intense situations. The following example is from the Adult Children's Support Group:

About six months before, Barry had told the group "I hope that my mother dies before she gets much worse." Other group members expressed shock that he wished his mother dead. The discussion was very emotional and very beneficial as it allowed group members to eventually acknowledge the mixed emotions involved with caregiving and the death of a parent. Barry's statement allowed the more fearful members to begin discussing this taboo topic and help to normalize it. Since then, the group appeared more comfortable raising the issue. A new group norm was formed allowing the following interchange:

Barry: I'll tell you something. My mother is really deteriorating fast. She has really gone downhill in the last year. I just hope that she dies soon. I had to see my father get so bad he was in a nursing home. It was horrible. I don't want my mother to go through that. I hope she just dies before I have to see her leave her home.

Caroline: One thing I worry about is the guilt I'll have when my mother dies. My friend's mother just died and she gave me some advice I want to share with everyone. She told me that whatever I do I should never, ever lose my patience with my mother or I will always regret it after my mother dies. At my friend's mother's funeral she was sobbing over her casket begging for forgiveness because of all the times she was so impatient with her. I don't want that to be me.

Albert: I always tell myself not to act that way with my mother but hard as I try I lose it with her.

Group worker: What do people think of the advice Caroline's friend gave her?

Barry: It's something to keep in mind.

Group worker: Is it possible to never lose your patience? Ed, what do you think?

Ed: No, it's not possible unless you're Mother Theresa.

(Everyone laughs.)

Ed: I lose my patience a lot. My mother can be infuriating. But I try my best. That's all I can do. And Barry, I agree with you. I am hoping that my mother dies before she gets to the point that she doesn't know anyone.

Barry: And one great thing about Alzheimer's is that my mother never remembers anything. I may be feeling guilty and she's already forgotten that anything happened.

Caroline: That's really a blessing, isn't it?

Again it was Barry who raised the issue of death but the group seemed more comfortable discussing it. Caroline gave advice that the group worker believed set totally unrealistic expectations but was not challenged. Instead, it immediately raised feelings of guilt. The group worker asked for members' reactions in order to get an exchange of views, eventually calling on Ed to give his opinion. Ed used humor to disagree allowing other group members to develop their own point of view. Even Caroline might be tempering the advice she had just given. This brief example of group dialectical process illustrates how even the most serious topics begin to be aired and examined.

CONCLUSION AND IMPLICATIONS

As the number of family caregivers continues to explode, those working in programs designed to support them need to be knowledgeable and sophisticated about their needs. The marker framework of caregiving is one useful tool in marketing caregiver support groups, selecting group members and in helping members throughout their caregiving careers. Increasing public awareness of family caregiving issues is likely to result in earlier consideration of support groups. Familiarity with the opportunities and challenges which earlier contacts raise enables group workers to make the most of these contacts. Success in identifying the servable moment (Montgomery & Kosloski, 2001) or point at which caregivers are most receptive to information and services will help to target marketing efforts.

Although the marker framework can be a valuable tool, it is not a formula applicable to all in the same way. Many different factors affect the caregiving career of every individual. Differences based on culture, relationship, gender, nature of illness, family dynamics, and personal experiences are just a few which have an impact. Markers can be reached in different orders, simultaneously, or some never reached at all. The skills of the group worker in assessing both the group and its members are primary. The marker framework is an aid in that assessment.

Finally, further exploration is needed regarding how best to serve caregivers through support groups. Is it more helpful for members to be segregated according to relationship, gender, length of caregiving, and/ or nature of illness? Will members find it easier to bond with and relate to caregivers going through similar experiences? Or is it possible that a more diverse group of caregivers leads to a richer experience and deeper understanding of caregivers with differing points of view? Research into these questions should incorporate the marker framework to help analyze whether differing factors impact the markers in predictable ways. This information will assist in deciding whether to form more specialized support groups and help workers anticipate differences in reactions in group members whether spoken or unspoken. When members reach caregiving markers, the need for both emotional support and concrete information on community resources and entitlements becomes especially important. Group workers with a firm grounding in both areas will be most helpful.

REFERENCES

Arno, P.S., Levine, C., & Memmott, M.M. (1999). The economic value of informal caregiving. *Health Affairs*, 18 (2), 182-188.

Bass, D.M., McCarthy, C., Eckert, S., & Bichler, J. (1994). Differences in service attitudes and experiences among families using three types of support services. *The American Journal of Alzheimer's Care and Related Disorders & Research*, May/ June, 28-38.

Batt-Leiba, M.I., Hills, G.A., Johnson, P.M., & Bloch, E. (1998). Implications of coping strategies for spousal caregivers of elders with dementia. *Topics in Geriatric Rehabilitation*, 14 (1), 54-62.

Brody, E., Saperstein, A.R., & Lawton, M.P. (1989). A multi-service respite program for caregivers of Alzheimer's patients. *Journal of Gerontological Social Work*, 14, 41-74.

Collins, C., Stommel, M., King, S., & Given, C.W. (1991). Assessment of the attitudes of family caregivers toward community services. *The Gerontologist*, 31 (6), 756-761.

Cummings, S.M. (1996). Spousal caregivers of early stage Alzheimer's patients: A psychoeducational support group model. *Journal of Gerontological Social Work*, 26 (3/4), 83-98.

Dobrof, J., & Ebenstein, H. (2004). Family caregiver self-identification: Implications for health care and service professionals. *Generations*, Winter, 33-38.

Dobrof, J., Zodikoff, B.D., Ebenstein, H., & Phillips, D. (2002). Caregivers and professionals partnership: A hospital based program for caregivers. *Journal of Gerontological Social Work*, 40 (1/2), 23-40.

Feder, J., Komisar, H.L., & Niefeld, M. (2000). Long-term care in the United States: An overview. *Health Affairs*, 19 (3), 40-56.

Feinberg, L.F., & Ellano, C. (2000). Promoting consumer direction for family caregiver support: An agency-driven model. *Generations*, Fall, 47-53.

Fredman, L., & Daly, M.P. (1998). Enhancing practitioner ability to recognize and treat caregiver physical and mental consequences. *Topics in Geriatric Rehabilitation*, 14 (1), 36-44.

Garland, J., Jones, H., & Kolodny, R. (1973). A model for stages of development in social work groups. In Saul Bernstein (Ed.), *Explorations in group work*. Boston: Milford House, Inc., 17-71.

Gottlieb, B.H., & Johnson, J. (2000). Respite programs for caregivers of persons with dementia: A review with practice implications. *Aging & Mental Health*, 4 (2), 119-129.

Henry J. Kaiser Foundation, Harvard School of Public Health, United Hospital Fund of New York & Visiting Nurse Service of New York (2002, June). *The wide circle of caregiving, Key findings from a national survey: Long-term care from the caregiver's perspective*. Author.

Houts, P.S., Nezu, A.M., Nezu, C.M., & Bucher, J.A. (1996). The prepared family caregiver: A problem-solving approach to family caregiver education. *Patient Education and Counseling*, 27, 63-73.

Junn-Krebs, U. (2003). Group work with seniors who have Alzheimers or Dementia in a social adult program. *Social Work with Groups*, 26 (2), 51-65.

Kaye, L.W., & Applegate, J.S. (1993). Family support groups for male caregivers: Benefits of participation. *Journal of Gerontological Social Work*, 20 (3/4), 167-185.

Kelly, K. (1997). Building aging programs with online information technology. *Generations*, Fall, 15-18.

Kelly, T. B., & Berman-Rossi, T. (1999). Advancing stages of group development theory: The care of institutionalized older persons. *Social Work with Groups*, 22 (2/3), 119-138.

Kurland, R., & Salmon, R. (1998). *Teaching a methods course in social work with groups.* Alexandria, VA: Council on Social Work Education, 35-69; 131-146.

Levine, C. (1999). The loneliness of the long-term caregiver. *The New England Journal of Medicine*, 340 (20), 1587-1590.

Liu, K., Manton, K.G., & Aragon, C. (2000). Changes in home care use by disabled elderly persons: 1982-1994. *Journal of Gerontology: Social Sciences*, 55B (4), S245- 253.

McCallion, P., & Toseland, R. (1995). Supportive group interventions with caregivers of frail older adults. In M. Galinsky & J. Shopler (Eds.), *Support groups: Current perspectives on theory and practice.* Binghamton, NY: The Haworth Press, Inc., 11-25.

Monahan, D.J. (1994). Caregiver support groups: Efficacy issues for educators. *Educational Gerontology*, 20, 699-714.

Montgomery, R.J.V., & Borgatta, E.F. (1989). The effects of alternative support strategies on family caregiving. *The Gerontologist*, 29, 457-464.

Montgomery, R.J.V., & Kosloski, K.D. (2001). Change, continuity, and diversity among caregivers. U.S. Administration on Aging website: www.aoa.gov/aoacarenet/Rmontgomery.html.

National Alliance for Caregiving & AARP (1997). *Family caregiving in the U.S.: Findings from a national survey.* Washington, DC: Author

Northen, H., & Kurland, R. (2001). *Social work with groups.* (3rd ed.). New York: Columbia University Press, 238-436.

Prigerson, H.G. (2003). Costs to society of family caregiving for patients with end-stage Alzheimer's disease. *The New England Journal of Medicine*, 349 (20), 1891-1892.

Sanders, S., & Corley, C.S. (2003). Are they grieving? A qualitative analysis: Examining grief in caregivers of individuals with Alzheimer's disease. *Social Work in Health Care*, 37 (3), 35-53.

Schiller, L.Y. (1995). Stages of group development in women's groups: A relational model. In R. Kurland, & R. Salmon (Eds.), *Group work practice in a troubled society: Problems and opportunities*, Binghamton, NY: The Haworth Press, Inc., 117-138.

Schulz, R., Mendelsohn, A.B., Haley, W.E., Mahoney, D., Allen, R.S., Zhang, S., Thompson, L., & Belle, S.H.. (2003). End-of-life care and the effects of bereavement on family caregivers of persons with dementia. *The New England Journal of Medicine*, 349 (20), 1936-1942.

Schulz, R., O'Brien, A.T., Bookwala, J., & Fleissner, K. (1995). Psychiatric and physical morbidity effects of dementia caregiving: Prevalence, correlates, and causes. *The Gerontologist*, 35, 771-791.

Shenk, D. (2001). *The forgetting, Alzheimer's: Portrait of an epidemic*. New York, NY: Doubleday.

Shulman, L. (1999). *The skills of helping: Individuals, families, and groups* (4th ed.). Itasca IL: F.E. Peacock.

Steinberg, D.M. (1997). *The mutual-aid approach to working with groups: Helping people help each other*. Northvale, NJ: Jason Aronson, Inc.

Toseland, R. (1995). *Group work with the elderly and family caregivers*. New York: Springer Publishing Company, Inc., 141-152.

Telephone Caregiver Support Groups

Tamara L. Smith, PhD (candidate)
Ronald W. Toseland, PhD
Victoria M. Rizzo, PhD
Michele A. Zinoman, MSW, PhD (candidate)

SUMMARY. This article describes the Telephone Support Group Model (TSG), a 12-week group work intervention designed to provide support to caregivers. Telephone support groups provide assistance for hard-to-reach caregivers. Caregivers who are traditionally deterred from face-to-face groups because of social constraints, geographic isolation, or physical limitations, or who are homebound because of the needs of the care recipient, are more able to participate in telephone support. A description of the 12 TSG sessions is provided. Two case examples are provided that illustrate the therapeutic benefits of TSG for caregivers and their families. Adaptations necessary for conducting telephone groups, and the advantages and disadvantages of this type of group

This project was supported in part by a grant to the Senior Services of Albany, Inc. and the Institute of Gerontology, University at Albany, number 90-CG-2549, from the Administration on Aging, Department of Health and Human Services, Washington, DC 20201. Grantees undertaking projects under government sponsorship are encouraged to express freely their findings and conclusions. Points of view or opinions do not, therefore, necessarily represent official Administration on Aging Policy.

[Haworth co-indexing entry note]: "Telephone Caregiver Support Groups." Smith, Tamara L. et al. Co-published simultaneously in *Journal of Gerontological Social Work* (The Haworth Social Work Practice Press, an imprint of The Haworth Press, Inc.) Vol. 44, No. 1/2, 2004, pp. 151-172; and: *Group Work and Aging: Issues in Practice, Research, and Education* (ed: Robert Salmon, and Roberta Graziano) The Haworth Social Work Practice Press, an imprint of The Haworth Press, Inc., 2004, pp. 151-172. Single or multiple copies of this article are available for a fee from The Haworth Document Delivery Service [1-800-HAWORTH, 9:00 a.m. - 5:00 p.m. (EST). E-mail address: docdelivery@haworthpress.com].

work, are discussed. Strategies for evaluating the quality of telephone interventions are also described. *[Article copies available for a fee from The Haworth Document Delivery Service: 1-800-HAWORTH. E-mail address: <docdelivery@haworthpress.com> Website: <http://www.HaworthPress.com> © 2004 by The Haworth Press, Inc. All rights reserved.]*

KEYWORDS. Support groups, elderly, caregiving, telephone groups, teleconferencing, technology

More than 50 million people are providing care to a chronically ill spouse, relative, or friend in the United States (National Family Caregivers Association, 2003). Caregiving for an older, chronically ill individual is a time-consuming job that frequently leads to the depletion of financial resources and to the compromised physical and mental health of the caregiver (Eisdorfer, Czaja, Loewenstein, Rubert, Arguelles, Mitrani, & Szapocznik, 2003; Brodaty, Green, & Koschera, 2003). Often, the caregiver becomes isolated from friends, family, and social activities. This isolation, and a lack of time for self-care, can result in the caregiver feeling overwhelmed, burdened, and stressed (Eisdorfer, Czaja, Loewenstein, Rubert, Arguelles, Mitrani, & Szapocznik, 2003; Bauer, Maddox, Kirk, Burns, & Kuskowski, 2001; Tebb & Jivanjee, 2000; Call-Theide, Finch, Huck, & Kane, 1999).

Support group interventions that incorporate social networking, counseling, problem-solving skills, and educational training have been found to reduce caregiver stress and burden while increasing the caregiver's psychological well-being (Cooke, McNally, Mulligan, Harrison, & Newman, 2001; Gallagher-Thompson, Lovett, Rose, McKibben, Coon, Futterman, & Thompson, 2000; Toseland, McCallion, Smith, Huck, Bourgeois, & Garstka, 2001). However, it can be difficult for caregivers to attend face-to-face groups because they live in rural areas, lack transportation or have conflicting responsibilities such as the inability to leave the care recipient at home alone (Galinsky, Schopler, & Abell, 1997; Glueckauf & Loomis, 2003; Martindale-Adams, Nichols, Burns, & Malone, 2002; Rosswurm, Larrabee, & Zhang, 2002). Some caregivers may also experience social discomfort from attending face-to-face support groups because of cultural and socioeconomic differences between themselves and other caregivers in the group, or because they have personality traits that make them uncomfortable talking in face-to-face groups (McKenna & Green, 2002).

Moreover, most caregiver programs described in the literature have been offered to middle-class white caregivers and have not served poor, culturally diverse, or isolated caregivers (see, for example, Toseland & Rossiter, 1989; Toseland & McCallion, 1997; Toseland, McCallion, Smith, Huck, Bourgeois, & Garstka, 2001). In an effort to offer support groups to caregivers who may not otherwise have access to these services, pioneering researchers and clinicians over the last decade have implemented support groups for caregivers by means of the telephone (Galinsky, Schopler, & Abell, 1997; Martindale-Adams et al., 2002; McCarty & Clancy, 2002). The aims of this article are to (1) review the empirical literature regarding the advantages and disadvantages of using telephone support groups with caregivers, (2) discuss the design and implementation of a telephone support group that was created to offer all caregivers, including minority caregivers, the opportunity to join a telephone support group in Upstate New York, and (3) describe the implementation factors that should be considered when running a telephone support group.

The existing literature regarding the use of telephone support groups suggests that they have certain advantages over face-to-face groups (Galinsky, Schopler, & Abell, 1997; McKenna & Green, 2002; Smokowski, Galinsky, & Harlow, 2001; Toseland & Rivas, in press). For example, caregivers find telephone support groups more accessible and more convenient than face-to-face groups. They increase participation because members do not have to leave their homes to attend. The use of telephone technology has been shown to overcome barriers to attendance. Telephone groups provide greater privacy, which in turn can reduce stigma for caregivers. A greater sense of anonymity not only reduces the anxiety associated with disclosing personal information, but also helps to facilitate communication between the worker and the group members (Colon, 1996; Lester, 1995).

Because members' identities are masked and because differences that are not salient to the purposes of the group are less likely to interfere with interaction, members are more willing to interact with one another and to share issues that are taboo in in-person groups. The security that participation is anonymous can lead to increased disclosure, truthfulness, and closeness among members. Moreover, these groups help to empower caregivers while decreasing feelings of burden. This is done by providing them with the necessary information regarding access to community resources, caregiving skills training, and emotional support (Martindale-Adams et al., 2002; McFarland & Sanders, 2000; Lindsey-Davis, 1998).

Telephone groups can help to serve hard-to-reach populations. For example, caregivers who are homebound due to their caregiving responsibilities, or because of their own physical or mental disabilities, can attend a telephone support group (Chase, Goodman, & Pynoos, 1990). Telephone groups can also be used to reach out to a variety of caregivers who do not attend face-to-face support groups, including geographically isolated, male, and minority caregivers and caregivers with time constraints (Martindale-Adams, Nichols, Burns, & Malone, 2002; McFarland & Sanders, 2000).

Because the time commitment for a telephone conversation is less constricting than traveling to a support group, telephone groups can be assembled more quickly than face-to-face groups. In scheduling these groups, caregivers have fewer time constraints because of the flexibility of making a telephone call as opposed to traveling to a group. In addition, conducting support groups over the telephone may reduce transportation costs and facility costs related to renting meeting space or having refreshments at the meetings. Finally, side conversations are more likely to be averted in telephone groups, and caregivers stay on-task more easily than in face-to-face groups (Galinsky, Schopler, & Abell, 1997), though additional research is needed to confirm this.

Despite the advantages of telephone groups, there are some limitations. For example, given that these groups are conducted in the privacy of the caregiver's home, the leader has no eye contact or visual cues to interpret. The lack of non-verbal and visual cues may change the group dynamics. The lack of visual cues also dictates that the leader take an active role to ensure that all participants are involved and enabled to take part in group sessions (Lester, 1995; Martindale-Adams et al., 2002; Nokes, Chew, & Altman, 2003).

Potential technological disadvantages should also be considered. These include the physical strain of being on a telephone for the duration of the group meeting, difficulty in hearing over the phone for hearing-impaired individuals, the fatigue that can occur with frail and/or elderly caregivers (Stein, Rothman, & Nakanishi, 1993; Wiener, Spencer, Davidson, & Fair, 1993), the risks of being disconnected during the group session, and the lack of third-party reimbursement (Nokes, Chew, & Altman, 2003; McCarty & Clancy, 2002). Unlike face-to-face support groups, there is no socialization time for members occurring either before or after the meeting. The group session is abruptly ended with the disconnection of the call (Rounds, Galinsky, & Stevens, 1991).

Cost can be another disadvantage of leading telephone support groups. Conference call equipment is expensive, and multiple telephone lines are needed if an organization sponsoring telephone groups decides to purchase its own equipment to make conference calls without going through an outside vendor. This is optimal for large agencies or organizations that intend to organize many telephone groups. If the equipment and telephone lines are not purchased, then a conference call provider must be used. Internet teleconference providers are less expensive than teleconference providers that do not use the Internet, but currently it still costs about $50 per meeting to connect eight members for an hour using an Internet provider if the organization sponsoring the group pays the telephone charges incurred by all group members. Prices may be reduced in the future, however, as Internet telephone technology becomes more widely available. Even considering these potential disadvantages of telephone support groups, this mode of support can be an invaluable tool for helping caregivers, and may be especially helpful for meeting the needs of vulnerable, hard-to-reach populations.

THE TELEPHONE SUPPORT GROUP (TSG) MODEL

The TSG model is an adaptation of a face-to-face support group model that has been evaluated in a number of studies in the past decade (see, for example, Toseland, Blanchard, & McCallion, 1995; Toseland, McCallion, Smith, Huck, Bourgeois, & Garstka, 2001). The face-to-face intervention consisted of eight weekly sessions that were each two hours in length.[1] In order for the telephone format to be successful, the original model was modified and the TSG model consisted of 12 weekly telephone support group meetings of one hour and 15 minutes. To address the possible fatigue that can occur with longer phone calls, the length of each meeting was decreased from two hours in the original model to one-hour phone calls, with an additional 10- to 15-minute connection time before the meeting, to address the possible fatigue that can occur with longer phone calls. We added four additional sessions to ensure that all of the content in the original face-to-face group model was included in the adapted telephone model. The additional connection time before each meeting was necessary in the TSG model because (1) some members were not always available the first time they were called and (2) the group leader needed one to two minutes to individually connect and greet each member using the Internet teleconferencing service provider we selected.

The TSG model consists of three components (emotion-focused coping, problem-solving coping, and support) that are interwoven into each group meeting. The first component, emotion-focused coping, occurs during the first half of each weekly TSG meeting. Emotion-focused coping is based on the Stress Inoculation Training (SIT) developed by Meichenbaum and colleagues (Meichenbaum, 1977, 1985; Meichenbaum & Cameron, 1983). Emotion-focused coping utilizes strategies such as: didactic teaching, cognitive restructuring, perspective taking, relaxation training, self-monitoring and self-instruction. To the extent possible these strategies are implemented in three phases: (1) conceptualization and assessment, (2) skill acquisition and rehearsal, and (3) application and follow-through. The social worker leading the group describes the techniques, and encourages members to practice them in each telephone support group meeting, and between meetings.

The second component, problem-focused coping, is introduced and practiced during the second half of each weekly meeting. Problem-focused coping starts by having members identify pressing problems that they would like to work on in the group. A six-step, problem-solving model is used: (1) describe the problem as specifically as possible, (2) identify the things that cause and sustain the problem and that interfere with your attempts to resolve it, (3) group generation of alternative problem-solving strategies without evaluation, (4) examine the advantages and disadvantages of each option, (5) develop a plan of action, and (6) evaluate the action plan and modify as needed.

In order for problem-solving to be an effective tool to help caregivers, the social worker leading the group should: (1) encourage all group members to identify a pressing problem they would like to address throughout the course of the TSG program and help them reframe problems that appear unsolvable so that productive problem-solving can occur, (2) encourage the participation of all group members in developing possible solutions for pressing problems, and (3) be familiar with community resources and services available to participants as possible avenues of finding solutions to their problems.

The third component of the TSG model, support, is interwoven throughout the two previously mentioned components of each group meeting. The group leader helps members to: (1) ventilate their feelings and concerns, (2) provide and receive empathetic understanding, (3) share different ways of coping with caregiving (i.e., peer helping), (4) feel hopeful about their situation, (5) play useful and meaningful roles by sharing their knowledge and experience with others in the group, and (6) provide peer models of how to effectively deal with stressful caregiving issues. To help group members develop supportive relationships beyond the TSG program, group members are assigned a telephone buddy whom they are encouraged to call in between group meetings to talk about their caregiving issues, to discuss the skills they are learning, and to receive support as they work on the goals they have identified to address their pressing problem. The mutual aid approach (Steinberg, 1997) is widely used in group work practice. By interweaving support into every meeting, telephone support groups such as the TSG Model demonstrate this approach to group work.

As is customary in short-term psychoeducational approaches to group work, each of the 12 weekly TSG meetings covers a preset agenda. Time is set aside each week for a brief didactic presentation by the social worker about emotion and problem-focused coping strategies, and some time is designated for discussion and practice. Group members are given participant workbooks to use between meetings to reinforce the skills learned each week. These workbooks include meeting agendas and accompanying written materials, a resource list for caregivers, a caregiver's bill of rights, and homework exercises (Rizzo & Toseland, 2003). Table 1 outlines the content of the meetings in the TSG model.

As shown in Table 1, the first half of each weekly meeting begins with the conference call hook-up. In face-to-face groups, small talk is initiated as members arrive, and the conference call hook-up is treated in this same manner. The group leader prevents long silences from occurring during the hook-up period by initiating interactions and by encouraging members to talk with each other. After the initial hook-up period, the group leader begins with a brief overview of the prior week's meeting, and asks members if they have any questions. This is followed by a "check-in" with group members regarding their between-meetings assignments, which include contacting their telephone buddies and practicing the skills they have learned in the group that are helping them progress toward their self-identified goals. The remainder of the first half of the meeting is devoted to an educational presentation of an emotion-focused coping strategy. The topics of these presentations are listed in Table 1. More detailed descriptions of the content are included in the training manual for the TSG program (Rizzo & Toseland, 2003).

The second half of each meeting focuses on the problem-solving component of the TSG model. The group leader asks participants if one of them would like to identify a pressing problem she/he would like to focus on with group input. Using the problem-solving steps outlined earlier in this paper, the group leader facilitates a problem-solving dis-

TABLE 1. Description of TSG Weekly Meetings

Meeting #1	**Meeting #2**	**Meeting #3**
Conference Call Hook-up (15 minutes)	Conference Call Hook-up (15 minutes)	Conference Call Hook-up (15 minutes)
Introductions (20 minutes)	Brief Overview of the First Meeting (5 minutes)	Brief Overview of the Second Meeting (5 minutes)
Purpose, Format, & Goals of the Group (10 Minutes)	Check-in Progress with Telephone Buddies (10 minutes)	Check-in Progress with Telephone Buddies (10 minutes)
Housekeeping and Group "Rules" (10 Minutes)	Cargivers Reactions to Caring for Care Recipients' Illnesses (10 minutes)	Problem Solving/Taking Time for Oneself (25 minutes)
Telephone Buddies (10 Minutes)	Impact of Chrionic Illness (15 minutes)	Care Recipients Reactions to Chronic Illness (20 minutes)
Problem Solving/Taking Time for Oneself (15 minutes)	Problem Solving/Taking Time for Oneself (15 minutes)	
Between Meetings (5 minutes)	*Between Meetings (5 minutes)*	*Between Meetings (5 minutes)*

Meeting #4	**Meeting #5**	**Meeting #6**
Conference Call Hook-up (15 minutes)	Conference Call Hook-up (15 minutes)	Conference Call Hook-up (15 minutes)
Brief Overview of the Third Meeting (5 minutes)	Brief Overview of the Fourth Meeting (5 minutes)	Brief Overview of the Fifth Meeting (5 minutes)
Coping Skills (25 minutes)	Check-in About Progress Toward Goals (10 minutes)	Check-in About Progress Toward Goals (10 minutes)
Problem Solving/Taking Time for Oneself (25 minutes)	Taking Time for Oneself (20 minutes)	Informal Supports (20 minutes)
	Problem Solving/Taking Time for Oneself (20 minutes)	Problem Solving/Taking Time for Oneself (20 minutes)
Between Meetings (5 minutes)	*Between Meetings (5 minutes)*	*Between Meetings (5 minutes)*

Meeting #7	**Meeting #8**	**Meeting #9**

Meeting #7

Conference Call Hook-up
(15 minutes)

Breig Overview of the Sixth
Meeting (5 minutes)

Services and Resources
(20 minutes)

Problem Solving/Taking
Time for Oneself
(20 minutes)

Between Meetings
(5 minutes)

Meeting #8

Conference Call Hook-up
(15 minutes)

Brief Overview of the
Seventh Meeting (5 minutes)

Check-in About Progress
Toward Goals (15 minutes)

Deep Breathing
(10 minutes)

Problem Solvingf/Taking
Time for Oneself
(25 minutes)

Between Meetings
(5 minutes)

Meeting #9

Conference Call Hook-up
(15 minutes)

Brief Overview of the Eighth
Meeting (5 minutes)

Check-in About Progress
Toward Goals (10 minutes)

Deep Breathing
(5 minutes)

Progressive Muscle
Relaxation (15 minutes)

Problem Solving/Taking
Time for Oneself
(20 minutes)

Between Meetings
(5 minutes)

Meeting #10

Conference Call Hook-up
(15 minutes)

Brief Overview of the Ninth
Meeting (5 minutes)

Check-in About Progress
Toward Goals (10 minutes)

Progressive Muscle
Relaxation (15 minutes)

Problem Solving/Taking
Time for Oneself
(25 minutes)

Between Meetings
(5 minutes)

Meeting #11

Conference Call Hook-up
(15 minutes)

Breif Overview of the Tenth
Meeting (5 minutes)

Check-in About Progress
Toward Goals (10 minutes)

Self-Talk (20 minutes)

Problem Solving/Taking
Time for Oneself
(20 minutes)

Between Meetings
(5 minutes)

Meeting #12

Conference Call Hook-up
(15 minutes)

Brief Overview of the
Eleventh Meeting
(5 minutes)

Self-Talk, Perspective
Taking, and Cognitive
Imagery (20 minutes)

Using Strategies Selectively
(20 minutes)

Evaluation and Wrap-up
(15 minutes)

cussion with the group members. In earlier group sessions before the members have much practice in the use of this problem-solving technique, they will often identify problems that cannot be solved. For example, a group member may say her pressing problem is her spouse's advanced dementia. Group members and the group leader would be hard pressed to identify possible solutions for this problem. To avoid identifying unsolvable problems, it is important that the group leader reframe problems so that effective problem solving can occur. For example, the caregiver's identification of her spouse's advanced dementia as a problem can be reframed to a problem such as not being able to leave her spouse alone for safety reasons. This re-formed problem could be alleviated with home care or respite care so the caregiver could have some time for herself. Following problem solving, the group leader reinforces the tasks to be accomplished in-between meetings, such as contacting telephone buddies and practicing new skills learned during the group session.

THE TSG MODEL GROUP LEADER

The telephone support group program (TSG) for spouse and adult child caregivers of the frail elderly we describe here is currently being evaluated in a demonstration project jointly sponsored by a school of social welfare and a non-profit community agency with a long history of serving caregivers of the frail elderly. The project is funded by the United States Administration on Aging. The TSG program leader for this project is a master's degree social worker. She is receiving ongoing clinical supervision and training for treatment integrity purposes from a clinical social worker with nine years of experience working with chronically ill older adults and their families.

Social workers are ideally suited to lead TSG programs because their training is focused on the person-environment fit. Furthermore, social work clinical practice taking place in host agencies that typically serve elderly clients requires social workers to develop care coordination and case management skills that are well-suited for this intervention. However, the TSG program could be delivered by any clinician from an allied discipline (i.e., psychology, educational counseling, and nursing) who is familiar with how to work with chronically ill older adults and their families. The clinician best suited to lead these groups is one who has: (1) experience with short-term psycho-educational group work approaches (Toseland & Rivas, in press), (2) familiarity with the theoretical underpinnings of a stress and coping framework, particularly the work of Lazarus and Folkman (1984), (3) knowledge of problem-solving casework models, such as Reid's (1997) task-centered approach, and (4) experience working with caregivers of frail older persons.

Workers leading TSG programs should not do so in isolation. We recommend that they receive weekly clinical supervision. This supervision should focus on adherence to the original TSG protocol, and the specific problems, issues and concerns experienced by caregiving participants. Optimally, the weekly support groups are audiotaped by the group leader for review by the supervisor. It is important to note that participants' informed consent is necessary to do this in any counseling situation. The supervisor should provide the group leader with ongoing feedback about his/her leadership skills and ability to deliver the intervention as intended, strategies for keeping meetings on task, and consultation to address any significant concerns and problems, such as the disclosure of elder abuse, that may arise during group meetings.

CASE EXAMPLES

In order to illustrate the therapeutic benefits of telephone support groups for caregivers and their families, two brief case examples are presented, one from the third meeting of a telephone support group that is being conducted for children who are caring for a parent, and the other from the fourth meeting of a group for spouses caring for a disabled partner. The first case example is taken from the problem-solving portion of meeting three.

Case Example One–Mrs. A

Social Worker: We've now reached the problem-solving portion of our group today. So far, Calvin and Betty have presented problems in our previous sessions. Who has a problem that they would like to resolve this week? (extended silence)

Mrs. A: The problem that I would like to resolve this week is how to deal with my mother's constant demands. From the minute I wake up to the moment that I go to bed, she asks me to do things for her. She makes me so mad that I just want to leave. Sometimes I find myself saying things I don't mean. Then I feel so guilty.

Social Worker: Most of us are familiar with each other's voice by now, but it still might be helpful to mention first names once before we start to speak.

Mrs. A: I'm Millie with the problem.

Mr. C: I'm Dan. I know how you feel. My mother lives downstairs from me and she is constantly calling for me to come down and get her something. By the end of the day, I have no energy left to do the things that I want to do. I get so frustrated that sometimes I refuse to go down. Or, I don't answer the phone. Then I feel terrible.

Social Worker: So Millie, the problem you would like to deal with is how to more effectively manage the demands your mother makes on you. It sounds like others in the group are also dealing with this same problem. What I am also hearing is that this prevents you from taking care of yourself and doing the other things you need to do with your life? Am I capturing the problem accurately?

Mrs. A: Yes, that's it exactly.

Social Worker: Is everyone else clear about Millie's problem so we can do some brainstorming?

All Group Members: Yes.

Miss B: This is Jane. Have you thought about using home health aides to help care for your parents? I know that this has helped me in dealing with my father's constant need for care.

Mrs. A: That would never work. Who would pay for it?

Social Worker: Remember, in order to solve a problem we need to be open to the solutions that are offered. I know it's hard, Millie, but during the brainstorming your job is to listen to all possible solutions before we decide what ones you might like to try.

Mrs. A: Thanks for reminding me. I forgot. It's hard not to respond right away.

Mr. C: (laughs) Remember! I had the same problem last week.

Social Worker: You did fine. This is a skill that takes some practice. Does anyone else have any other suggestions?

Miss B: My mother qualified for home care services under Medicaid. I could explain how this works.

Mrs. D: This is Shirley. What about your family? I thought that you said that you had a brother and a sister?

Mrs. A: They never offer to help . . . I guess I could ask them. But, I don't know if my mother would ever let a stranger in the house.

Miss B: If your family cannot help, then you should see about home health aides. You could even stay in the house in the beginning to let your mom get comfortable.

Social Worker: Two suggestions have been made. First, that Millie consider home care for her mom. Second, that she ask her family to help. Does anyone else have any suggestions?

Mr. C: I don't have a new suggestion, but I'd like to say a little more about family help. When my mom came to live with my wife and me, I never thought to ask my sister to help. But then my wife encouraged me to ask her to come stay with my mom on some Saturday evenings so we could get some time together alone. I told my wife no way. I can't ask her. She'll just say no. But when I did ask her I was surprised. She was happy to help. I had just thought that since she said mom couldn't live with her that this meant she wouldn't help, but I was wrong. Now, my mom spends two weekends a month at my sister's and she comes to our house one evening a week to make her dinner and to visit so we can go out. It has helped a lot.

Miss B: Yeah, sometimes we assume people will know we want them to ask us if we need help, but we need to tell them what we need. I don't always do this myself.

Social Worker: That is an excellent point. (The social worker asks if anyone else has suggestions and reviews the possible solutions that were presented in the brainstorming.)

Social Worker: Millie, do any of the solutions sound like they might work for you?

Mrs. A: I just don't see home care as an option. My mom really doesn't like strangers in the house and I just think having them there would make things worse than they already are.

Miss B: You might be surprised if you ask her about it.

Mrs. A: No, I know my mom and this wouldn't work. My brother and his wife do live down the street and they both just retired. But I'm afraid to ask them to help because they had all these plans to travel in their motor home and visit places they've dreamed of.

Mr. C: Millie, didn't you have plans for what you want to do? I mean why should you have to take care of your mother all the time and your brother gets to have no responsibility. That doesn't seem fair. Has he said he wouldn't help?

Mrs. A: No, and sometimes his wife will ask if she can help and I don't even know what to ask her for help with.

Social Worker: Okay, this is a start. Millie, you said your mom makes constant demands on you all day. What could your brother and his wife do to make these demands more bearable? What would make the situation better for you?

Mrs. A: I don't know.

Mr. C: You know, my wife and I find my mom much easier to deal with now that my sister comes over and we get some time away. My mom is still difficult, but we can handle it better because we get time alone.

Social Worker: Do you think this would help, Millie? Getting some time away from your mom.

Mrs. A: Actually, before my mom needed so much help, I used to play Bingo on Tuesday nights with my friends at our church. I really miss it.

Miss B: Do you think your brother would stay with your mom? Could you ask him?

Mrs. A: I guess I could. The worst thing he could do is say no.

Social Worker: Do you think this is something you can do before we meet again and report back to us on how it went?

Mrs. A: I could try.

The social worker then reviews the problem-solving techniques that the group used to help Mrs. A identify a solution to the problem that she is willing to try out.

Case Example Two–Coping Skills

The next excerpt is from the eleventh meeting of a group for spouse caregivers. This portion of the meeting illustrates members helping each other to use coping skills.

Mrs. L: Lately, I feel as though my husband pretends to need me every time I am getting ready to leave the house. Just yesterday I was going to my friend's house for a cup of coffee across the street. As soon as I put my coat on, he began to ask me to help him. I got so mad at him I began to yell and then my chest got tight and I began to have trouble breathing. I just don't know what to do anymore . . .

Mrs. M: I used to feel this way all the time, but I've been using the breathing exercises we learned and they help me to calm down when I feel this way. (no response from the group)

Social Worker: Mary (Mrs. L), I think that Laura (Mrs. M) was addressing that to you. Have you tried the deep breathing exercise we practiced?

Mrs. L: Yes, it has helped a little but I find it hard to remember to do it right then.

Mrs. M: I practiced it every day for awhile. Now when he makes me mad I just stop and do some breathing exercises before I scream at him. I'm calmer and I don't create more problems with my screaming.

Mrs. S: I thought that I was the only one who ever felt this way.

Social Worker: What way is that?

Mrs. S: Well, lately I just want to scream every time I have to take my husband to the bathroom.

Mr. F: I find it so hard to keep a good outlook. It seems as though I never get out, but you know, I did get a commode for the bedroom so that I do not have to walk my wife down the hall every time she needs to use the bathroom. Maybe this could help you with your problem. My insurance pays for it.

Mrs. Q: Remember during our last group meeting we talked about my going away for the weekend for the first time in over a year. I was so nervous leaving my husband at respite, but I feel like a new person. I really think that I am going to set aside a weekend a month just to stay home and relax . . . Has anyone else thought about this?

Social Worker: This is such a good point. It is so important for each of you to take some time for yourselves. Let's talk about why we all need to focus on our own well-being and ways in which we can actually do this.

As the group continues, the social worker facilitates a discussion on ways members have been taking care of themselves, and what more they could be doing to take care of themselves. The worker's role in the discussion is to empower members by encouraging them and "giving them permission" to take time out for themselves.

ADAPTATIONS FOR TELEPHONE SUPPORT GROUPS

To ensure a smooth introduction to participating in telephone groups, the group leader should be knowledgeable and comfortable with the technology. It can be helpful to practice using the technology for the first time with colleagues or friends. The conference calls should be made as user-friendly as possible for participants, with a clear explanation of how the technology will work, and what to do in the event of any technical difficulties. Finally, the group leader should always have a back-up plan if technical difficulties do arise. This may include planning with members that they will be called back later the same day or on a different day.

To successfully facilitate a telephone support group, the telephone support group leader often needs to be more active than in face-to-face groups. In go-rounds, for example, the leader has to indicate who should introduce themselves next, as the visual cues of a circle or nonverbal cues, such as a nod from the group leader, are not visible. During interactions, the group leader may find it necessary to make connections between members by directing questions from one group member to other members. Also, the group leader often has to repeat questions asked by group members because members may not have expected to respond to particular questions. The group leader should have participants identify themselves each time they communicate, particularly in early group meetings when members are not familiar with each other's voices, and at the beginning of later group meetings, until the leader is sure that members remember each other's voices. Even in later group meetings it is sometimes difficult to distinguish people with similar voices. Therefore, certain members may need to identify themselves more frequently. Without the benefit of seeing who is speaking, it can be confusing to follow a conversation if members do not identify themselves before speaking.

Structure is also more important in telephone groups than in face-to-face groups. Structure helps members to stay organized and on-topic and allows them to anticipate what will occur next during group meetings. Also, information and materials that were used in group meetings were sent out well ahead of time and included an agenda and necessary materials for each meeting.

Because there are no non-verbal cues, it is essential for the group leader to prompt members to clarify statements and to give clear feedback to one another during the telephone calls. The group leader should also check to ensure that members' emotional reactions are understood correctly, and to make sure that these are clear to all group members.

In addition, it helps to have members anticipate problems that are inherent in telephone conference calls, while at the same time appreciating the benefits of the medium. Problems include missed cues and interruptions that caregivers may experience during group meeting times. Missed cues are easily handled by repeating phrases, clarifying, making connections, and asking for feedback. Interruptions such as the doorbell ringing or a caregiving chore, while infrequent, do occasionally occur. We have found that caregivers are good about letting other members know if they have to leave the conversation for a period of time. They also are good about letting members know when they return to the teleconference call. Still, it is important to tell members in the first meeting to let other members know if they have to leave the conversation and to announce when they rejoin the group. Other group members understand that members may be called away for caregiving responsibilities, but notification of a brief absence is important to avoid confusion. We have found that it is also helpful to check at the beginning of meetings whether any member is expecting an unusual but unavoidable disruption, such as the delivery of an appliance. Notification of a possible disruption tends to minimize its impact when it does occur during a meeting.

EVALUATION

At the completion of a telephone support group, it is advisable to ask individual group members about their experiences in the group. This allows for modifications to be made to existing protocol, and it offers leaders feedback on their abilities to run the group smoothly. If possible, someone other than the group leader should administer these evaluations in private, so that group members can honestly assess their experiences.

In our demonstration project, group members were called by a member of the evaluation team after they completed the 12-week TSG program, and were asked a series of questions pertaining to their participation. For example, we asked participants whether they were interrupted during the phone calls, whether their time spent on the phone conflicted with their caregiving responsibilities, whether they used the participant workbook, what sections of the workbook they found most helpful, how they would rate the intervention compared to a face-to-face intervention, and what they liked most and least about the group. As a result of asking these questions, we found that the majority of caregivers did not have any disruptions while they were on the telephone. When disruptions did occur, however, the most common reasons included the pressing needs of the care recipient, or the needs of a family member or other person who was helping to provide care while the caregiver attended the telephone group meeting. These interruptions seldom impacted the caregiver's ability to benefit from the group experience. Caregivers indicated that a disrupted telephone support group call was preferable to no support. Caregivers also expressed that they rarely felt that their time on the telephone interfered with performing their caregiving responsibilities.

Respondents who participated in the first few support groups stated that they sometimes needed to help the care recipients unexpectedly during the phone call. Because of this feedback, we were able to suggest that participants in later groups ask a family friend or neighbor to visit with the care recipient during the telephone group time. After we made this suggestion, interruptions declined.

Overall, members indicated that they enjoyed participating in the telephone support groups. Participants cited as reasons for their enjoyment the short-time commitment, the friendliness of the other participants and the group leader, the sense of bonding that participants felt to other caregivers by talking to one another about their problems, the opportunity to get information, the opportunity to hear other people's insights and how they handle problems, and the problem-solving com- ponent of the group. Overall, group members felt connected to other members of their group, providing preliminary evidence that the group reduced social isolation. The things that participants liked least about the group were: (1) no face-to-face contact, (2) hearing difficulties, (3) technological problems, and (4) the length of the meeting. It should be noted, however, that some respondents felt that the meetings were too long, whereas others thought that the meetings were too short.

The feedback that we received from participants helped us greatly to improve the quality of the intervention that we have been able to deliver to subsequent groups of participants. In response to comments made by group members who evaluated early group meetings, the group leader more frequently clarified communications and made more frequent connections between members. She more actively encouraged non-talkative participants to take an active role in the group. She changed the original internet telephone conference provider to one with a more reliable connection. Finally, she was more active in checking with members before the group began about who wished to be one of the earlier callers connected. Those with more stringent time constraints sometimes needed to be connected to the call as close to the official starting time as possible.

CONCLUSION

The use of telephone support group interventions for caregivers has increased over the past decade. Telephone caregivers support groups can provide assistance to isolated caregivers who are excluded from traditional support groups because of a lack of transportation, geographical distance, financial costs of attending a group, their inability to leave the care recipient alone, and their discomfort in traditional face-to-face support groups.

Future research on telephone support group interventions should include rigorous evaluations of these groups. Randomized control group studies, with a pretest/posttest design, are recommended to identify outcomes from these groups, and to compare the outcomes of these groups to face-to-face groups. Future research may also want to focus on the use of telephone support groups for specific subgroups of caregivers, such as long-distance caregivers, intergenerational caregivers, and caregivers providing care to care recipients with specific health problems, such as dementia or stroke.

NOTE

1. A manual for leading face-to-face caregiver support groups or for leading telephone caregiver support groups and workbook manuals for participants can be obtained by writing to Ronald Toseland, Institute of Gerontology, University at Albany, State University of New York, 135 Western Avenue. Albany, NY 12222.

REFERENCES

Bauer, M., Maddox, M., Kirk, L., Burns, T., & Kuskowski, M. (2001). Progressive dementia: Personal and relational impact on caregiving wives. *American Journal of Alzheimer's Disease and Other Dementias, 16* (6), 329-334.

Brodaty, H., Green, A., & Koschera, A. (2003). Meta-analysis of psychosocial interventions for caregivers of people with dementia. *American Geriatrics Society, 51,* 657-664.

Call-Theide, K., Finch, M., Huck, S., & Kane, R. (1999). Caregiver burden from a social exchange perspective: Caring for older people after hospital discharge. *Journal of Marriage & the Family, 61,* 688-699.

Chase Goodman, C., & Pynoos, J. (1990). A model telephone information and support group for caregivers of Alzheimer's patients. *The Gerontologist, 30* (3), 399-404.

Colon, Y. (1996). Telephone support groups: A nontraditional approach to reaching underserved cancer patients. *Cancer Practice, 4* (3), 156-159.

Cooke, D., McNally, L., Mulligan, K., Harrison, M., & Newman, P. (2001). Psychosocial interventions for caregivers of people with dementia: A systematic review. *Aging & Mental Health, 5* (2), 120-135.

Eisdorfer, C., Czaja, S., Loewenstein, D., Rubert, M., Arguelles, S., Mitrani, V., & Szapocznik, J. (2003). The effect of a family therapy and technology-based intervention on caregiver depression. *The Gerontologist, 43* (4), 521-531.

Galinsky, M., Schopler, J., & Abell, M. (1997). Connecting group members through telephone and computer groups. *Health & Social Work, 22* (3), 181-188.

Gallagher-Thompson, D., Lovett, S., Rose, J., McKibben, C., Coon, D., Futterman, A., & Thompson, L. (2000). Impact of psychoeducational interventions on distressed caregivers. *Journal of Clinical Geropsychology, 6* (2), 91-110.

Glueckauf, R., & Loomis, J. (2003). Alzheimer's caregiver support online: Lessons learned, initial findings, and future directions. *NeuroRehabilitation, 18,* 135-146.

Lazarus, R., & Folkman, S. (1984). *Stress, appraisal, and coping.* New York: Springer.

Lester, D. (1995). Counseling by telephone: Advantages and problems. *Crisis Intervention, 2,* 57-69.

Lindsey-Davis, L. (1998). Telephone-based interventions with family caregivers: A feasibility study. *Journal of Family Nursing, 4* (3), 1-16.

Martindale-Adams, J., Nichols, L., Burns, R., & Malone, C. (2002). Telephone support groups: A lifeline for isolated Alzheimer's disease caregivers. *Alzheimer's Care Quarterly, 3 (2),* 181-189.

McCarty, D., & Clancy, C. (2002). Telehealth: Implications for social work practice. *Social Work, 47* (2), 153-161.

McFarland, P., & Sanders, S. (2000). Educational support groups for male caregivers of individuals with Alzheimer's disease. *American Journal of Alzheimer's Disease and Other Dementias, 15* (6), 367-373.

McKenna, K., & Green, A. (2002). *Virtual Group Dynamics: Theory, research, and practice, 6* (1), 116-127.

Meichenbaum, D. (1977). *Cognitive behavior modification–An integration approach.* New York: Plenum.

Meichenbaum, D. (1985). *Stress inoculation training.* New York: Plenum.

Meichenbaum, D., & Cameron, R. (1983). Stress inoculation training: Toward a general paradigm for training coping skills. In D. Meichenbaum & M.E. Jaremko (Eds.), *Stress reduction and prevention* (pp. 115-154). New York: Plenum.

National Family Caregivers Association. Retrieved on December 14, 2003, from *http://www.nfcacares.org/.*

Nokes, K., Chew, L., & Altman, C. (2003). Using a telephone support group for HIV-positive persons aged 50+ to increase social support and health-related knowledge. *AIDS Patient Care STDS, 17* (7), 345-351.

Reid, W. (1997). Research on task-centered practice. *Social Work Research, 21*(3), 132-137.

Rizzo, V., & Toseland, R. (2003). *Telephone Support Group Program: A participant workbook.* Albany, NY: Institute of Gerontology, University at Albany, State University of New York.

Rosswurm, M., Larrabee, J., & Zhang, J. (2002). Training family caregivers of dependent elderly adults through on-site and telecommunications programs. *Journal of Gerontological Nursing,* July, 27-38.

Rounds, K., Galinsky, M., & Stevens, L.S. (1991). Linking people with AIDS in rural communities: The telephone group. *Social Work, 36* (1), 13-18.

Smokowski, P.R., Galinsky, M., & Harlow, C.K. (2001). Using technologies in group work, part II: Computer based groups. *Group Work, 13* 98 B 115.

Stein, L., Rothman, B., & Nakanishi, M. (1993). The telephone group: Accessing group service to the homebound. *Social Work with Groups, 16* (1/2), 203-215.

Steinberg, D.M. (1997). *The mutual-aid approach to working with groups: Helping people help each other.* Northvale, NJ: Jason Aronson, Inc.

Tebb, S., & Jivanjee, P. (2000). Caregiver isolation: An ecological model. *Journal of Gerontological Social Work, 34* (2), 51-72.

Toseland, R., Blanchard, C., & McCallion, P. (1995). A problem-solving intervention for caregivers of cancer patients. *Social Science and Medicine, 40,* 517-528.

Toseland, R., & McCallion, P. (1997). Trends in caregiving research. *Social Work Research, 21,* 3, 154-165.

Toseland, R., & Rivas, R. (In press). *An introduction to group work practice* (5th ed.). Needham Heights, MA: Allyn & Bacon.

Toseland, R., & Rossiter, C. (1989). Group interventions to support family caregivers: A review and analysis. *The Gerontologist, 29,* 438-448.

Toseland, R., McCallion, P., Smith, T., Huck, S., Bourgeois, P., & Garstka, T. (2001). Health education group for caregivers in an HMO. *Journal of Clinical Psychology, 57* (4), 551-570.

Wiener, L., Spencer, E.D., Davidson, R., & Fair, C. (1993). National telephone support groups: A new avenue toward psychosocial support for HIV-infected children and their families. *Social Work with Groups, 16* (3), 55-71.

Elderly Parents of Adults
with Severe Mental Illness:
Group Work Interventions

Harriet Goodman, DSW

SUMMARY. Seriously mentally ill adults frequently require assistance from their parents over many years. As parents age, they confront the dual challenge of caregiver demands and the need to cope with their own aging. Support groups for aging parents are a key component of social support for families that care for a mentally ill family member. This paper presents evidence of the value of support groups for elderly caregivers, through both current literature and a case example that provides a window into the strength of group work to help this vulnerable population of caregivers. *[Article copies available for a fee from The Haworth Document Delivery Service: 1-800-HAWORTH. E-mail address: <docdelivery@ haworthpress.com> Website: <http://www.HaworthPress.com> © 2004 by The Haworth Press, Inc. All rights reserved.]*

KEYWORDS. Support groups, psychoeducational groups, multi-family groups, elderly adults, caregivers, seriously mentally ill adults, caregiver burden, caregiver reward, stigma

---

[Haworth co-indexing entry note]: "Elderly Parents of Adults with Severe Mental Illness: Group Work Interventions." Goodman, Harriet. Co-published simultaneously in *Journal of Gerontological Social Work* (The Haworth Social Work Practice Press, an imprint of The Haworth Press, Inc.) Vol. 44, No. 1/2, 2004, pp. 173-188; and: *Group Work and Aging: Issues in Practice, Research, and Education* (ed: Robert Salmon, and Roberta Graziano) The Haworth Social Work Practice Press, an imprint of The Haworth Press, Inc., 2004, pp. 173-188. Single or multiple copies of this article are available for a fee from The Haworth Document Delivery Service [1-800-HAWORTH. 9:00 a.m. - 5:00 p.m. (EST). E-mail address: docdelivery@haworthpress. com].

The onset of serious mental illness occurs in late adolescence, at a point in a person's life when they would normally become emancipated and begin living on their own. Instead, seriously mentally ill adults frequently become dependent on their families and require continued assistance from their parents over the course of many years (Milliken, 2000). Of the 10 million people in the United States with a diagnosis of serious mental illness, an estimated 4.8 million have a serious and persistent mental illness. Of this group, approximately one-third live with their families on an ongoing basis (Psychiatric Services, 1997). The caregiving burdens for these families are longstanding, lasting over years of worry, guilt, grief, isolation, and insufficient help from mental health professionals (Biegle & Schulz, 1999).

Parents have assumed a greater burden of care for their chronically mentally ill children since the 1950s and 1960s spawned the community mental health movement and deinstitutionalization (Mowbray & Holter, 2002). People who once were treated in hospitals now receive care in the community. However, enhanced civil rights for people with serious mental illness means they are not required to use community services. In fact, they may avoid contact with community mental health providers. When clients are hospitalized, their stays are shorter. Clients may return to the community and their families with more severe problems than in the past. The community mental health system remains strained, uninviting, and case managers are often unable to decrease clients' dependency on the family (Biegel & Schulz, 1999).

Groups have provided support and education for parents of people with serious mental illness for decades (Galinsky & Schopler, 1995). Educational groups have helped parents become less critical and overprotective, resulting in better outcomes for their adult children in the community (McLean et al., 1982). Support groups for parents have had a normalizing effect for members who share the social stigma ascribed to families touched by serious mental illness. Family members themselves recognized limitations of the formal mental health system to address their many unmet needs and, as a result, group initiatives have grown out of their own efforts to organize. The National Alliance for the Mentally Ill (NAMI), with its long history of peer-led self-help groups, has served as ballast against perceived burdens mental health providers have placed on family members over the years.

This article will trace how four decades of theory, policy, and practice in treating seriously and persistently mentally ill people have affected parent caregivers (McCallion & Toseland, 1995). Then, the author will review issues in family function, and the burdens and rewards of family caregiving for chronic mental illness, focusing on changing needs of caregivers as they age. Finally, the article will discuss various group interventions available for aging parent/caregivers of adult children with major mental illness, concluding with a case example that highlights issues in implementing groups for this vulnerable population.

THE CONTEXT FOR PARENTS CARING
FOR MENTALLY ILL ADULT CHILDREN

In recent years, following policies to deinstitutionalize people with severe mental illness, the majority of seriously mentally ill people live in the community. However, community mental health care has not kept pace with the progress of deinstitutionalization. Consequently, the burden of care for patients often falls to their parents who are middle-aged or elderly (Milliken, 2000). Community-based systems of support for adults with serious mental illness remain an unfulfilled goal. Many barriers to care remain. Mentally ill clients need services such as housing, job training, or social skills training, but they are not widely available (Biegel & Schulz, 1999). Parents, who may already be approaching middle age when a child first receives a diagnosis of a severe mental disorder, can look forward to years of caregiving.

Assisting one family member by another is a normative and pervasive activity. But traditional tasks go beyond the bounds of usual care when the parent/caregiver faces the expenditure of time and energy over an extended time (Biegel & Schulz, 1999), and when stigmatized illness generalizes to the family caregivers (Lefley, 1989). In addition, while parents assume responsibility for their mentally ill adult children, neither the legal system, mental health practitioners, or the adult children recognize parental rights. Milliken (2000) calls this condition "disenfranchisement," that is, parents lack the rights they feel necessary to care for their adult children.

ISSUES FOR AGING CAREGIVERS

The Burdens of Caregiving

The concept of caregiving "burden" has been divided into two descriptive categories, "objective" and "subjective" burdens. Objective burdens are practical hardships, such as providing assistance in daily activities, financial hardship due to medical bills, or disruption of family and social life. Occupational disruption or role changes also constitute objective burdens. Subjective burdens are psychological distress including stress, tension, anger, worry, guilt, or shame (Lefley, 1989; Bulger et al., 1993; Schwartz & Gidron, 2002).

Protracted caregiving for someone with severe mental illness exacts a physical, financial and psychological toll. Maintaining a child with mental illness can be expensive, and parents will pay personally for extra treatment and medications that medical insurance does not cover. The illness itself may precipitate profligate spending or poor money management skills, with parents covering costs. Parents may also incur substantial financial losses in time taken off from paid work, or may stop working altogether, to meet the patient's needs (Millekin, 2001). In situations where only one caregiver is available to the patient, that caregiver is significantly more likely to lack employment, adding to financial difficulties, and is also more vulnerable to social isolation (Harvey & Burns, 2003).

Parents have a difficult time managing the subjective or emotional burdens of caregiving. Parents have described their experiences as caregivers as "living with sorrow, anguish, and constant worry," and "living with guilt and shame" (Pejlert, 2001). They express frustration about their inadequacies, resulting in tension, poor health, and guilt. Coping with the overwhelming emotional stress is more difficult to manage than coping with day-to-day crises or problems. Parents ride an emotional "roller-coaster" that correlates with the vicissitudes of the illness trajectory. Milliken (2001) describes a repeated cycle of guilt, denial, hope, despair, anger, and depression that both mothers and fathers experience as "disenfranchised grief."

PARENT BLAMING AND STIGMATIZING FAMILIES

Parents' interactions with the mental health system are often negative and reinforce a caregiver's identity as a "disenfranchised parent" or worse. A number of outdated psychodynamic theories attribute schizophrenia, in particular, to family interactions. Theories such as "marital schism and skew," the "double-bind" hypothesis, and the "schizophrenogenic mother" branded parental behaviors as the source of severe mental illness (Milliken, 2000). Empirical research does not support these theories of etiology. Critics have pointed out their tautological nature (Torrey, 1995), and the current scientific literature attributes psychotic disorders to physiological forces that produce neurochemical abnormalities in the brain (Rubin et al., 1998). However, some mental health practitioners continue to view family members as toxic agents, particularly in schizophrenia and the roundly unsupported stereotype of the schizophenogenic family (Lefley, 1989).

Outdated practitioner views about family culpability persist, even though new evidence indicates that treatment modalities that cause parents to feel they are to blame for causing and perpetuating their children's psychotic disorders are not only ineffective, but may actually harm the person with mental illness (Rubin et al., 1998). In a study of social work students and practitioners, Rubin et al. (1998) found that although most practitioners recognize that biological factors are important in the etiology of serious mental illness, approximately half of their practitioner respondents continued to believe parents bear responsibility for their children's mental illness. Consequently, for these social workers, the aim of therapy with parents is to get them to recognize their culpability.

Social workers are not the only professionals who need to learn to support the efforts of parents caring for mentally ill children in the community. Pejlert (2001) conducted a phenomenological study of parent caregivers. Their experiences with the mental health system, and nurses in particular, were long and dismal; mental health workers blamed parents for their child's illness. As parents continued to devote themselves to caring for their children, their actions were questioned as over-involved or dysfunctional. Nurses were unwilling to share planning, leading to what the researcher labeled a "culture conflict" between the family system and the care system (Pejlert, 2001).

In the face of the tenacity with which social workers and other mental health workers hold on to discredited theories, current evidence-based treatments promote very different practices for families and patients. They support family members, educate them about psychiatric disorders, and foster the development of support networks. Under the rubric of psychoeducation, they strive to build alliances between family members and practitioners. Perhaps most importantly, they not only absolve parents of blame, but also recognize parents are secondary victims of a biologically-based illness (McFarlane, 2002).

While there has been much discussion of stigmatization of mentally ill people, family members also experience stigma. Parents may find themselves isolated when friends and neighbors erect social barriers. When people with psychotic disorders display socially offensive behavior, the family may experience further isolation (Lefley, 1989). The guilt expressed by many parents of children with severe mental illness intensifies when society sends the message that they are, in fact, guilty parties in the illness of their child.

AGING CAREGIVERS AT RISK

The role of caregiver may be undesired and has the potential to create an at-risk population among aging parents whose own mental health may deteriorate from the stress and sorrow associated with the psychotic disorder of their child (Lefley, 1989). Aging caregivers confront the dual challenge of continuing caregiver demands and the need to cope with the consequences of their own aging (Seltzer et al., 1995). Elements of objective and subjective burdens are specific to mental illness. The patient fails to carry out age-appropriate functions with consistency, mirrored by the cycles of exacerbation and remission of symptoms. Parents encounter stressors such as interactions with emergency services or police, involuntary commitment procedures that pit parents against their children, and difficulties locating alternative care in the community. Parents are often frustrated, confused, and humiliated in their encounters with mental health service providers (Lefley, 1989).

Risks that family caregivers of all ages experience may put aging parents at special risk when they care for an adult psychotic child. Abuse and assault, financial losses, unprovoked aggression, and the impact of stress on psychological and physical health highlight the vulnerability of the aging caregiver. Elderly parents of chronic patients are concerned about what will happen to the patient "when they are gone" (Lefley, 1989). Given the widely recognized failed promise of community-based mental health programs for persons with serious mental illness (Biegel & Schulz, 1999), these concerns may be well-founded.

As early as 1987, Lefley drew attention to the large number of elderly caregivers of people with serious mental illness. She recognized the problem this would cause for the mental health service system, as large numbers of aging caregivers were becoming frail and would die. Older caregivers experience strain, embarrassment, and resentment when the mentally ill family member is disruptive. Many older caregivers give care at the expense of their own health and well-being (Lefley, 1987), and the impact of caregiving stressors can have profound effects on the health of the aging parents, their ability to care for their child and, indeed, on the health-care system in general (Lebowitz & Light, 1996). Declining health also puts aging caregivers at greater risk for depression (Seltzer et al., 1995).

When compared with aging mothers caring for adult children with mental retardation, those caring for adults with mental illness experience more profound problems. They have more symptoms of depression, and their coping strategies are less likely to buffer the stress they experience as caregivers. The caregiving experience is less predicable, since the cyclical nature of behavior problems and other symptoms creates uncertainty about how their adult child will react each day. These parents have endured years of interaction with an unresponsive mental health system, and they tend to rely less on problem-focused coping strategies, perhaps because of the limited control they have experienced over years of contact with the mental health system (Seltzer et al., 1995).

When Cook and Lefley (1994) looked at caregiving issues over the life span, they recommended that older parents receive help with estate planning and provision of services after the parent's death. However, older parents of adult children with mental illness apparently are not making plans, leading Hatfield (2000) to conduct a study that combined qualitative and quantitative methods to identify obstacles parents encountered in planning, as well as the degree to which they had completed plans. In this study, 96% of the parents in the study were members of the National Alliance for the Mentally Ill. Only 18% of the respondents had completed plans for their children. The parent caregivers expressed extreme anxiety about the future, and they did not think that professionals would be helpful with end-of-life decision-making. However, when elderly parents did turn to the mental health system, two-thirds found it helpful. Providers clearly need to be more proactive engaging aging caregivers in planning for their children's future (Hatfield, 2000; Duvdevany & Keren, 2002).

Lefley and Hatfield (1999) suggest preparing both caregivers and patients for parental aging and eventual loss to help both overcome psychological barriers for establishing continuing care management. One specific resource available in some states is The Planned Lifetime Assistance Network established through the National Alliance for the Mentally Ill, which provides lifetime assistance to disabled people whose parents are no longer able to provide care (Lefley & Hatfield, 1999; National Alliance for the Mentally Ill, 2004).

The Rewards of Caregiving

Recently, researchers have explored the rewards for family care-givers of severely mentally ill people (Bulger et al., 1993; Heru, 2000; Schwartz & Gidron, 2002), family resiliency (Marsh & Lefley, 1996), and an "atmosphere of competence" in families (Johnson, 2004). These studies indicate that some parents may experience rewards as caregivers for their mentally ill children. They challenge mental health profession-als to expand the conception of the family experience of mental illness to include resiliency and competency. Schwartz and Gidron (2002) re-ported that their subjects found considerable gratification as caregivers. Satisfaction from fulfilling their parental sense of duty was particularly prominent. Despite the heavy strain of caring for a mentally ill, depend-ent child, parents felt that caregiving had important emotional rewards.

Few researchers have studied the concept of caregiver reward for parents of people with severe mental illness. However, three findings about caregiver reward are particularly important for group work practi-tioners with aging caregivers. First, family intimacy appears to be corre-lated with reward and may help explain why some families cope better than others do. Second, older caregivers have less negative affect than younger ones. Finally, support groups may be a significant component of successful treatment for aging caregivers (Heru, 2000).

Bulger and colleagues found in his study of 60 adults that family caregivers experienced gratification and intimacy with their adult chil-dren, and in many cases more gratification than burden. Since all sub-jects in their study were recruited from a support group organization, this association suggested groups might be a powerful component in re-ducing burden and maximizing reward (Bulger et al., 1993). Although Schwartz and Gidron (2002) do not infer a relationship between the gratification expressed by their sample, the fact that their subjects came exclusively from support group participants is notable. It appears that support group participation may enhance coping skills, reduce burden, and allow for acknowledgment of reward (Heru, 2000).

Cook and Heller (1999) tested the positive association between de-creased subjective caregiver burden and support group participation. Their positive findings were minimal and confounded by greater reports of depression, strain, and stressors from people who attended the groups. Group attendees also rated their children as much less inte-grated in the community as the control group parents (Cook & Heller, 1999). Regrettably, some report that intervention studies of support groups as compared to other mental health interventions have used the weakest designs (Biegel & Schulz, 1999). However, more recently, Saunders (2003), in her extensive review of the literature on families living with severe mental illness, reports strong evidence of the value of support groups; they are a key component of social support for families that provide care for a family member with severe mental illness.

GROUP INTERVENTIONS FOR ELDERLY CAREGIVERS OF SERIOUSLY MENTALLY ILL CHILDREN

Support Groups

Support groups for family caregivers of adults with serious mental illness have been described for decades (Winefield et al., 1998; Heller et al., 1997; Walsh et al., 1996; McLean et al., 1982). Group programs provide social support and expand the social networks of families caring for mentally ill children. Support groups are able to give parents a venue to express their desire for better mental health services, acquire accurate information regarding their children's illness, and gain respect from professional mental health workers (Saunders, 2003).

Nevertheless, caregivers come to support groups for many more reasons: to share experiences and coping strategies, exchange information, and gain access to new resources. Groups also provide education, validation of painful decisions, and understanding and companionship from people who share their situation. Other group members understand the pain, know the system, have information about resources, and are more likely than natural kinship networks to provide an empathic system of care. Support group membership can also provide an entry point for parents to assume action-focused coping to gain better control over their lives (Lefley, 1997). Social support received by group members can be associated with members acquiring more information outside of the group (Heller et al., 1997). For elderly caregivers, these benefits of support group participation can be an opportunity to begin exploration of end-of-life planning for their children's future.

Some support groups for family members caring for people with serious mental illness use guides for group leaders. The National Alliance for the Mentally Ill (NAMI) has long experience with peer-led support groups. The rationale for peer-led groups is located in NAMI's commitment to family empowerment, recognition of shrinking mental health dollars, and demands for cost effectiveness (Cook & Heller, 1999).

The organization currently offers a set of key structures and group processes for facilitators to use in common. The National Alliance for the Mentally Ill considers group facilitators key to making support groups a positive and productive experience for members. They promote and sponsor co-leadership training for facilitators to address issues such as group structure, member roles, workers' use of self, and problem-solving. The National Alliance for the Mentally Ill promotes their group model for both seasoned and less-experienced facilitators (National Alliance for the Mentally Ill, 2003).

Psychoeducation and Multifamily Groups

The efforts of advocacy organizations, such as the National Alliance for the Mentally Ill, have pressed professional mental health providers to recognize the potential for a partnership with family members of seriously mentally ill patients. The insistence of family members that they wanted to work towards helping their children was the backdrop against which combined psychoeducational and support groups developed. Psychoeducational groups are a potent method to increase caregivers' knowledge of their child's serious and persistent mental illness and to learn better behavior management skills at home (McCallion & Toseland, 1995). As neuroscience and behavioral interventions proved valuable to mentally ill people, parents and professionals alike benefited from understanding the developing knowledge base of the etiology of mental disorders, and psychopharmacological and behavioral interventions (McFarlane, 2002).

Multifamily groups in the treatment of severe mental illness have a four-decade history. They originally began in hospital settings to address ward management problems. More recently, the groups combine a psychoeducational component with a therapeutic social network that supports families and people with mental illness. As with support groups generally, these interventions help reduce the shame and guilt family members experience, and promote relief and heightened morale among participants. The additional feature is to help participants gain information about the mental illness that is affecting the family. Ultimately, the groups have four major functions. First, they establish an alliance between families and knowledgeable, empathic professionals. Then they provide current research-based information about the mental illness. Third, they present guidelines for illness management, and finally, they help participants practice solving problems created by the illness (McFarlane, 2002).

Multifamily psychosocial group applications cover a range of specific disorders: schizophrenia, bipolar disorder, major depressive disorder, and obsessive-compulsive disorder (McFarlane, 2002). Some multifamily psychoeducational groups are highly predetermined. Social group workers will find these curriculum-driven initiatives place the mental health providers at the center of the process and diminish the power of group members to find strengths in their historic caregiving role. Group workers should become involved in developing these programs, since they are easy to adapt to a curriculum-based format that would allow for more member control.

SPECIAL ISSUES IN GROUP WORK PRACTICE WITH ELDERLY CAREGIVERS: A CASE EXAMPLE

The following case example describes the experiences of a student intern assigned to work with a group of eight elderly women who were caregivers for their mentally ill children, "The Mother's Group." The interdisciplinary geriatric team originally created the group to provide the opportunity for mutual support in caring for their mentally ill children and, more ominously, to help members explore other interests or hobbies that would help them separate from their children. The student was appropriately alarmed that she was instructed not to reveal the second "purpose" to the group members, since the team was concerned the second goal would "scare members away":

> My supervisor instructed me to attempt to guide the group toward greater independence from their children and report to the team. I found it frustrating to try to move the group toward a goal they had no prior knowledge of and no interest in pursuing. The group's motivation and focus was not directed to achieving the same purpose as the one set out for them.

> The members had in common that they were all women, 65 years or older, caring for an adult child with severe mental illness. For them, the purpose of the group was to fulfill the need for support, normalize their intense feelings, alleviate their isolation, and find practical suggestions and advice. They were from diverse religious backgrounds.

As I got to know the group better, I realized that the progress notes written about the group by other workers failed to do justice to the unique dynamics inherent in the group. One point of interest that emerged over several months was the fear the members had of the use of the word "crazy." One session, a group member called another member "crazy" because she had given her mentally ill daughter a huge part of her savings to see a private dentist. The "crazy" member left the group early, whereupon, the name caller expressed her guilt and called the member during the week to apologize. The next session, I asked the group what it was about the word that they feared, but they denied my assertions and changed the topic several times.

Another session, a member came in and said she had seen the movie, *A Beautiful Mind*. The other members erupted in anger towards this member. They said they had enough mental illness to contend with on a daily basis, and they had no desire to hear about a movie on the subject. However, when I prodded them further, we had an open discussion where they revealed hidden fears of guilt and responsibility over having "given" their children a mental illness.

From my point of view, the group functioned well, and had for the past six years. But the prevalent view of the agency was that the members were "stuck in their ways." They were inflexible and unwilling to change or grow. At team meetings, workers laughed at how members would never change and didn't want to move beyond their problems.

Member recruitment and retention are considered problems for support groups for family members of persons with mental illness, since they may be reluctant to take the first step in joining (Walsh et al., 1996). Nonetheless, "The Mother's Group" proved to be a magnet for the elderly women who participated. Their attendance was remarkably stable, with an average of six members attending each session. Their participation was also active. Over the life of the group, they had clearly established norms that communicated sensitivity to the needs of the members to control their exposure to negative assaults from the community.

The irony of this group's survival is a testament to the shared needs of the members in the face of efforts on the part of professionals to override the meaning of the group in the women's lives. Unfortunately, it probably reflects professional attitudes the women experienced over a lifetime of care they provided for their mentally ill children. The women roundly rejected the "team's" covert purpose to try to have them explore hobbies that would enable them to separate from their children. Fortunately, the student group worker grew to understand the meaning the group had in these women's lives and was able to support their work.

Besides the risk she might have run in promoting undeclared purposes, this worker might never have challenged the members' reluctance to include direct content about mental illness in their meetings. Her ability to challenge the group members through a demand for work enabled them to explore feelings that are typical responses to caring for mentally ill children. The worker's ability to hear these expressions of guilt and grief made it possible for the women to express themselves, thus normalizing their feelings in an empathic system.

Because the group worker was a student, she could not confront the "team's" inappropriate group practice. However, as other students have communicated, a potent survival skill for group practitioners in settings unfamiliar with social group work principles is to focus on established group work skills and create a safe space in which the members can work (Goodman & Munoz, in press). The "team's" reactions to the women are an unfortunate reminder of the persistence of parent blaming and stigmatizing parents of children with mental illness. The fact that the members were elderly women only increased the probability the professional staff would stigmatize them.

CONCLUSION

This article has reviewed the context in which elderly parents of mentally ill children have experienced the profound impact of having a child diagnosed with a serious and persistent mental illness. An aged person involved in the care of a mentally ill child now has lived through a period of dynamic change in the systems that were supposed to provide support for their family. Unfortunately, that system failed to realize the promise of community treatment for their mentally ill child. Professionals who were supposed to care for their children saw parents as a part of the problem. Only recently are these mothers or fathers seen as having needs of their own or as possible partners in caring for their children, and the locus for including parents in care has occurred in advocacy, support, and psychoeducational groups.

Groups can profoundly shape the experience of elderly caregiving parents and their mentally ill children for the better. Lefley describes a support group she conducted for 10 years. She writes about a mother in the group who greeted newcomers with the words, "Just wait, you are in for a lifetime of hell!" This member had no friends, relatives, or social networks other than the group. Although a difficult member, when she developed breast cancer, it was the members who insisted she get treatment, helped her in her final days, helped her mentally ill son grieve his loss, and establish himself in a community residence (McFarlane, 2002, xi).

Aged caregivers of children with severe mental illness are a population at risk. The stress they experience in their roles makes them vulnerable to physical illness and depression. Their child's behaviors may result in physical injury or financial setbacks. They have real concerns about what will happen to their children when they are no longer alive.

The case example presented in this article supports the power of support groups to help elderly caregivers. It also reveals how groups can neutralize intractable negative attitudes on the part of some mental health professionals towards parents of people with serious mental illness. The power of this group to transcend the culture of the care system and establish its own culture of normalcy and acceptance provides a window into the strength of group work to help this vulnerable population of aging caregivers.

REFERENCES

Anderson, C. M., Griffin, S., Rossi, A., Pagonis, I., Holder, D. P., & Treiber, R. (1986). A comparative study of the impact of education vs. process groups for families of patients with affective disorders. *Family Process, 25*(2), 185-205.

Biegel, D. E., & Schulz, R. (1999). Caregiving and caregiver interventions in aging and mental illness. *Family Relations, 48*(4), 345-354.

Bolzan, N., Smith, M., Mears, J., & Ansiewicz, R. (2001). Creating identities: Mental health consumer to citizen? *Journal of Social Work, 1*(3), 317-328.

Brennan, J. W. (1995). A short-term psychoeducational multiple-family group for bi-polar patients and their families. *Social Work, 40*(6), 737-743.

Bulger, M. W., Wandersman, A., & Goldman, C. R. (1993). Burdens and gratifications of caregiving: Appraisal of parental care of adults with schizophrenia. *American Journal of Orthopsychiatry, 63*, 255-265.

Cook, J. A., & Heller, T. (1999). The effect of support group participation on caregiver burden among parents of adult offspring with severe mental illness. *Family Relations, 48*(4), 405-411.

Cook, J. A., & Lefley, H. P. (1994). Age and family burden among parents of offspring with severe mental illness. *American Journal of Orthopsychiatry, 64*(3), 435-448.

Deal, W. P. (1998). *Outcomes Associated with Participation in a Family Education Program for Caregivers of Individuals with Serious Mental Illness.*

Dreier, M. P., & Lewis, M. G. (1991). Support and psychoeducation for parents of hospitalized mentally ill children. *Health and Social Work, 16*(1), 11-18.

Duvdevany, I., & Keren, N. (2002). Thought, consideration and future planning for out- of-home placement among caregivers of dependent adult children with psychiatric disabilities. *International Journal of Rehabilitation Research, 25*(3), 207-213.

Galinsky, M. J., & Schopler, J. H. (Eds.) (1995). *Support Groups: Current Perspectives on Theory and Practice.* New York: The Haworth Press, Inc.

Goodman, H., & Munoz, M. (In Press). Developing social group work skills to preserve best practice. *Social Work with Groups.*

Harvey, K., & Burns, T. (2003). Relatives of patients with severe mental disorders: Unique traits and experiences of primary, nonprimary, and lone caregivers. *American Journal of Orthopsychiatry, 73*(3), 324-333.

Hatfield, A. B. (2000). Helping elderly caregivers plan for the future care of a relative with mental illness. *Psychiatric Rehabilitation Journal, 24*(2), 103-108.

Heller, T., Roccoforte, J. A., Hsieh, K., Cook, J. A., & Pickett, S. A. (1997). Benefits of support groups for families of adults with severe mental illness. *American Journal of Orthopsychiatry, 67*(2), 187-198.

Heru, A. M. (2000). Family functioning burden, and reward in the caregiving for chronic mental illness. *Families, Systems and Health: The Journal of Collaborative Family Health Care, 18*(1), 91-104.

Johnson, E. D. (2004). The role of families in buffering stress in persons with mental illness: A correlational study. In K. R. Yeager & A. R. Roberts (Eds.), *Evidence-Based Practice Manual: Research and Outcome Measures in Health and Human Services* (pp. 844-857). London: Oxford University Press.

Lebowitz, B. D., & Light, E. (1996). The aging caregivers of psychiatric patients: Healthcare perspectives. *Psychiatric Annals, 26*(12), 785-791.

Lefley, H. P. (1987). Aging parents as caregivers of mentally ill adult children: An emerging social problem. *Hospital and Community Psychiatry, 38,* 1063-1070.

Lefley, H. P. (1989). Family burden and family stigma in major mental illness. *American Psychologist, 44*(3), 556-560.

Lefley, H. P. (1997). Synthesizing the family caregiver studies: Implication for service planning, social policy, and further research. *Family Relations, 46*(4), 443-450.

Lefley, H. P., & Hatfield, A. B. (1999). Helping parental caregivers and mental health consumers cope with parental aging and loss. *Psychiatric Services, 50*(3), 369-375.

Marsh, D. T., & Lefley, H. P. (1996). The family experience of mental illness: Evidence for resilience. *Psychiatric Rehabilitation Journal, 20*(2), 3-12.

Marsh, D. T., & Lefley, H. P. (2003). Family interventions for schizophrenia. *Journal of Family Psychotherapy, 14*(2), 47-68.

McCallion, P., & Toseland, R.W. (1995). Supportive group interventions with caregivers of frail older adults. In M. J. Galinsky & J. H. Schopler (Eds.), *Support Groups: Current Perspectives on Theory and Practice* (pp. 11-25). New York: The Haworth Press, Inc.

McFarlane, W. R. (2002). *Multifamily Groups in the Treatment of Severe Psychiatric Disorders.* New York: The Guilford Press.

McLean, C. S., Greer, K., Scott, J., & Beck, J. C. (1982). Group treatment for parents of adult mentally ill. *Hospital and Community Psychiatry, 33*(7), 564-568.

Milliken, P. J. (2001). Disenfranchised mothers: Caring for an adult child with schizophrenia. *Health Care for Women International, 22,* 149-166.

Mowbray, C. T., & Holter, M. C. (2002). Mental health and mental illness: Out of the closet? *Social Service Review,* 135-179.

National Alliance for the Mentally Ill (2002). Planned Lifetime Assistance Network. Retrieved May 20, 2004, from *http://www.nami.org/Content/ContentGroups/Helpline1/PLAN__Planned_Lifetime_Assistance_Network_.htm*

National Alliance for the Mentally Ill (2003). NAMI Support Group Program. Retrieved May 20, 2004, from *http://www.nami.org/Content/NavigationMenu/Find_Support/Education_and_Training/Education_Training_and_Peer_Support_Center/NAMI_Support_Group/NAMI_Support_Group_Program.htm*

Pejlert, A. (2001). Being a parent of an adult son or daughter with severe mental illness receiving professional care: Parents' narratives. *Health and Social Care in the Community, 9*(4), 194-204.

Pfeiffer, M. M. (2001). The other parent: A qualitative study of fathers of severely and persistently mentally ill adult children. Unpublished doctoral dissertation, Bryn Mawr College, Bryn Mawr, PA.

Pollio, D. E. (2002). The evidence-based group worker. *Social Work with Groups, 25*(4), 57-70.

Psychiatric Services (1997). New methodologies for estimating the prevalence of mental illness finds 10 million adults affected. *Psychiatric Services, 48*(9), 1216.

Rubin, A., Cardenas, J., Warren, K., Pike, C. K., & Wambach, K. (1998). Outdated practitioner views about family culpability and severe mental disorders. *Social Work, 43*(5), 412-422.

Saunders, J. C. (2003). Families living with severe mental illness: A literature review. *Issues in Mental Health Nursing, 24,* 175-198.

Schwartz, C., & Gidron, R. (2002). Parents of mentally ill adult children living at home: Rewards of caregiving. *Health and Social Work, 27*(2), 145-153.

Seltzer, M. M., Greenberg, J. S., & Krauss, M. W. (1995). A comparison of coping strategies of aging mothers of adults with mental illness or mental retardation. *Psychology and Aging, 10*(1), 64-75.

Torrey, E. F. (1995). *Surviving Schizophrenia* (3rd ed.). New York: Harper Collins.

Walsh, J., Hewitt, H. E., & Londeree, A. (1996). The role of the facilitator in support group development. *Social Work with Groups, 19*(3/4), 83-91.

Winefield, H., Barlow, J., & Harvey, E. (1998). Responses to support groups for family caregivers in schizophrenia: Who benefits from what? *Australian and New Zealand Journal of Mental Health Nursing, 7,* 103-110.

Seniors, Small Fry, and Song:
A Group Work Libretto
of an Intergenerational Singing Group

Miriam Cusicanqui, MSW
Robert Salmon, DSW

SUMMARY. The development and implementation of an intergenerational singing group starting from the idea for the program and including all stages of group development from the planning stage to the ending stage are described. The importance of clarity of purpose for activities is emphasized. Two age groups, seniors and children, come together to sing, and to establish relationships. While largely successful, the lack of knowledge and understanding of the group work approach on the part of some of the professional staff adversely influenced the outcome. Includes a summary of research about groups of this kind and a review of the relevant social group work literature. *[Article copies available for a fee from The Haworth Document Delivery Service: 1-800-HAWORTH. E-mail address: <docdelivery@haworthpress.com> Website: <http://www.HaworthPress.com> © 2004 by The Haworth Press, Inc. All rights reserved.]*

KEYWORDS. Seniors, elders, intergenerational program, purposeful use of activities, group work, stages of development, endings

---

[Haworth co-indexing entry note]: "Seniors, Small Fry, and Song: A Group Work Libretto of an Intergenerational Singing Group." Cusicanqui, Miriam, and Robert Salmon. Co-published simultaneously in *Journal of Gerontological Social Work* (The Haworth Social Work Practice Press, an imprint of The Haworth Press, Inc.) Vol. 44, No. 1/2, 2004, pp. 189-210; and: *Group Work and Aging: Issues in Practice, Research, and Education* (ed: Robert Salmon, and Roberta Graziano) The Haworth Social Work Practice Press, an imprint of The Haworth Press, Inc., 2004, pp. 189-210. Single or multiple copies of this article are available for a fee from The Haworth Document Delivery Service [1-800-HAWORTH, 9:00 a.m. - 5:00 p.m. (EST). E-mail address: docdelivery@haworthpress.com].

INTRODUCTION

This article discusses the development of an intergenerational singing group, which included children in elementary school and seniors
living in a residence run by a settlement house in New York City. The
idea for the program, the challenges to its development and implementation, and the stages of development as it evolved, will be described.
The purpose will be specified, and the obstacles that were encountered
will be highlighted.

EXPOSITION

I[1] am the coordinator of the CAPS (Community Achievement Project in
Schools), a dropout-prevention program in an urban public school. CAPS
is a grant-funded program of the settlement house. The program's primary
goal is to support elementary school children and help them adjust to the
school environment and remain in school. Students referred to the program
must meet the following criteria: poor attendance (10 or more absences),
poor academic progress, repeating the grade, behavior problems, living in
transitional housing, in foster care, or being at risk of foster-care placement.
Many children are eligible. Individual and group counseling are provided
as part of the effort to achieve this goal. Activity often is used as a tool in
the counseling process. Children share their life experiences and participate
in problem-solving through the arts, storytelling, and active listening. Parents also come together to support each other. The group counseling process helps the parents, who then feel more competent and empowered in
helping their children to become more integrated within the school community.

Since the school year lasts for only nine months, I often work in another program site during the summer months. During one recent summer, I worked at the senior residence of the settlement house. This
residence provided supportive housing and services to a group of elders
who had many of the physical and emotional problems associated with
people of advanced age and limited resources. Many were frail and
health-disabled. Some were wheelchair-bound, used walkers, and needed other forms of personal assistance. The population was diverse.
About 40 percent were Russian, about 30 percent African-American.
There was a substantial Latino population as well. Many of the members were supported totally by Social Security payments. Some were on

welfare. They had been referred to the residence primarily by hospitals and other agencies.

This experience gave me the opportunity to provide direct service to seniors and to learn more about what they had experienced in their long lives. It also gave me a greater understanding of their often courageous adaptation to difficult circumstances. Many of these elders had few extended family members, and I sensed their struggle to stay connected to the community. They often found companionship and a sense of belonging by participating in activities in the residence. One of these activities is a singing group. As my assignment to the residence came to an end, I explained to the elders that I would be returning to work with children in the program site at the school. Many of the seniors expressed interest in perhaps coming to the school to tutor or volunteer to read to students in the dropout-prevention program. I realized that they yearned to establish a relationship with children.

When I was in graduate school, as a group-work major, I had the opportunity to see an extraordinary film, "Close Harmony" (1981). This academy-award-winning documentary showed the process of bringing together two large groups: the members of a very active senior citizens' center and children from a private elementary school, to become an intergenerational chorus. Among other benefits, the film showed the power of program to dispel stereotypes and to strengthen the connection and bonding of participants in this joint activity.

The singing group at the senior residence, where I had worked during the summer, and the dropout-prevention program are both sponsored by the same settlement house agency. The agency's philosophy attests to the use of mutual aid as a way to create a sense of community and empowerment in all program participants. There is extensive use of music and the visual arts in the planning of the agency's overall program. Also, the philosophical framework of the agency encourages a high degree of awareness of advocacy and social action. Mattaini, Lowery, and Meyer (1998) attest to the historical framework of settlement houses as to the use of group work. "Groups were established for people to learn skills necessary to participate in their neighborhood and communities" and to "socialize the individual." The agency's current mission is in keeping with this statement. The director of the agency, a group worker himself, endorses the group work approach to practice in the agency. And so, I considered the possible connection between the singing group at the senior residence and the dropout-prevention program. An idea was born. The agency could create an intergenerational singing group.

The emotional need for a connection to children was expressed clearly to me by the seniors. I believed the children would be interested as well. Such a program clearly was in keeping with the philosophy of the agency. I turned to the selected research on such efforts and to the literature on activity in social work in order to help me in the exploration and development of such a program.

REVIEW OF SELECTED LITERATURE

Research

Negative attitudes toward the elderly develop early in childhood (Burke, 1981). "Many studies have shown that younger people often hold negative attitudes toward the elderly and view them as senile, isolated, helpless, lethargic, unproductive, and stubborn" (Pinquart, Wenzel, and Sorensen, 2000; also see Palmore, 1990). Others hold positive attitudes toward the elderly, describing them as wise advisors or caring grandparents (Hummert, 1993). Also, more specifically, Ward, Kemp, and Newman (1996) reported that the results of their study provided evidence that weekly singing between nursing-home residents with dementia and nursery-school children had beneficial effects on the psychological well-being of the elderly residents. Pinquart, Wenzel, and Sorensen (2000) stated that, "The usefulness of a superordinate, common goal and of intergenerational cooperation on attitude change was demonstrated by the elderly participants, whereas the children improved their attitudes toward the elderly regardless of the amount of intergenerational cooperation." Aday, Sims, McDuffie, and Evans (1996) reported positive effects of intergenerational interventions on children's attitudes over a time period of one-to-five years. Finally, in the conclusions drawn from one study, it was stated that the activity reported should stimulate the further implementation of intergenerational activities.

> Intergenerational group work offers learning for both the young and the old. Successful cooperation and support across generations can help to eliminate age stereotypes. This study showed that both generations benefit from such interventions. (Pinquart, Wenzel, and Sorensen, 2000)

Social Work Literature

Much has been written about the history of social work and of group work. There is no intention to repeat it all here. However, much of the history is so related to what evolved in the attempt to develop the intergenerational singing group, that a selected literature review will be offered. The use of activity in work with groups always has created some controversy, and historically there has been substantial debate about its place and use in the profession. In early use of activity, what the group did–the content–was emphasized. This was particularly important and was stressed during the time of the settlement house movement. However, ". . . The emphasis on content of a group had an adverse effect historically on group work's acceptance as a method of social work . . ." (Northen and Kurland, 2001, p. 259). During and following the 1930s, activity and its emphasis on *doing* had less status than the *talking* that was the domain of work with individuals. "The early thinking, which presumed a dichotomy between talking and doing, continues to fuel debates today" (Kurland and Salmon, 1998, p. 110).

Grace Coyle (1946), in her famous address at the National Conference of Social Work, stressed the two dimensions in good group work practice–the activity and the interplay of personalities that create the group work process. She said, in part:

> Program and relationship are inextricably intertwined. Social work method developed as we began to see that the understanding and use of human relations involved were as important as the understanding and use of various types of program.

A milestone in development of the use of program was the 1949 publication of *Social Group Work Practice* by Gertrude Wilson and Gladys Ryland. They stressed the value in play and games and were the first to focus on the importance of nonverbal content. Although they did not discuss the connection between what the worker did and why, their contribution led to several decades of discussion of the relationship between group work theory and the use of program content (see as examples: Trecker, 1955; Vinter, 1974; Middleman, 1968 and 1982; and Shulman, 1971).

> The intrinsic connection between the use of program and the purpose of social work became increasingly recognized and appreciated, at least "officially," by social work's national organization

and by group workers themselves, if not by social work practitioners generally . . . (Kurland and Salmon, 1998, p. 111)

However, group work's place in the curriculum started to decline in
the 1960s as the Council on Social Work Education began the effort to
shift to generalist practice. Curriculum standards stressed generic social
work practice. "In most such social work practice courses, little time
was devoted to specific beliefs, knowledge, and skills that were the hall-
mark of group work. The use of program and activity was generally ignored altogether (Kurland and Salmon, 1998, p. 112).

In quite astounding fashion, however, the use of program and activity
in group work practice has refused to disappear. It can be of great value
in work with groups, and practitioners young and old discover this–and
write about it. Some recent examples follow. Erica Schnekenburger
(1995) wrote "Waking the Heart Up: A Writing Group's Story," an article about a creative writing group she formed and led. The group had a
life of seven months, and "The story illustrates, by tracing the group's
life, the usefulness and value that collaborative poetry can hold in mental health settings" (p. 19). A brief excerpt from the article gives testi-
mony to its usefulness and power, and the role of the worker.

> One week, we wrote a poem about the writing group: "Paint a picture
> of the group. What are we doing?" Ramona, who was once so silent
> and sleepy, gave the first line in her raspy voice:
>
> *"Waking the heart up."*
>
> Henry contributed:
>
> *By putting the word on paper*
> *It is beautiful, like a rose.*
>
> And as I reflected on my work with this group, I thought, people
> are also like roses. Some open up quickly, some slowly, some
> never at all. They cannot be opened by another. All I can do is help
> cultivate and create an atmosphere that will make it safe to happen.
> And when it does, respect, appreciate, and admire. (p. 31)

Whitney Wright (1999) discussed the process and formation of a coed
teenage ceramics group and the use of activity. She described how purpose
fluctuates over the life of the group, with the activity taking precedence in

the beginning, the growth-oriented purpose taking precedence in the middle stage, and both purposes sharing importance in termination (p. 31). A selection from Wright's article points great attention to the importance of stages of development, and of the worker's role. It demonstrates the power of the group and skillful group work.

The following excerpt again illustrates the need for high worker controls. It also illuminates how commonalities play a vital role in the beginning stage.

> The members were having a difficult time maintaining an ideal wetness and thickness of their pots and controlling the pressure of their fingers on the clay. Jessica pushed too hard and broke through the edge of her bowl.
>
> *Jessica: Oh, I ruined it. I broke the side of my bowl. I hate this. I can't do this.*
>
> *Worker: It looks to me like something other than a bowl now. Can anyone think of what it looks like?*
>
> *Tyrone: It looks sort of like a pitcher.*
>
> *Worker: That's exactly what I was thinking.*
>
> *(Jessica's face lit up. She turned it into a pitcher. Two other members turned their bowls into pitchers, too.)*
>
> Since the activity-oriented purpose is emphasized in the beginning stage . . . deeper connections to members' feelings in the group, or life outside the group, were not included. If the example given had been taken from the middle stage, a discussion of the benefit of looking at potential positive outcomes of mistakes might have been prompted by Jessica's pitcher. (p. 39-40)

David Dinolfo (2004), a professional dancer as well as a social worker, described his work with a group of developmentally challenged adults. His efforts were designed to help group members experience feelings of leading, and following, in group movement exercises and in the development of greater confidence while leading. The purpose of the group was to promote increased awareness of multiple choices, and confidence in decision-making while dancing with others. The following excerpts are from his paper. They are examples of role, stages of development, and the importance of purpose.

> The worker (dancing with Robert) is following Robert's movement and then, without saying anything, he takes the lead. Robert follows without a hitch. The worker continues for a while and then asks the group what they have seen. Aaron immediately says he noticed that the worker had taken over the lead. Robert, who had been following, said he hadn't noticed. The worker said, "Sometimes it is very hard to tell who is leading when you are watching, and sometimes following, too."

> Aaron had been very astute to have noticed the switch and had been watching carefully. The worker then made pairs of the group while they practiced mirroring each other and used nonverbal cues to switch leaders. The worker watched. The pairs successfully mirrored each other for a long period of time without getting bored or losing concentration. The mirroring pairs switched leaders back and forth with a minimum of verbalization and with little conflict. The worker had never seen the group members work together with such concentration and without becoming distracted.

> One person in each pair was designated the leader, and the worker encouraged the leaders to move slowly so they could be followed. At a few points, the worker instructed them to change leaders. Dennis was a better leader than follower and seemed to enjoy this role. The other pairs were very lively. The lead pair did not only slow-moving but some fast, explosive type movement which the others were able to follow. When this is done well, it is sometimes difficult for an audience to know which is the leader, as happened here. The worker commented that even the facial expressions were mirroring one another–both broad grins and giggles.

> The mirroring exercise described above would not have been appropriate or effective in the beginning stage of this group. Trust was a necessary ingredient for the success of the mirroring exercise and occurred in the middle stage. A higher demand for competence and an ability to tolerate failure had been established. Also, I believe that an understanding on the part of group members regarding the purpose of the group and the decision-making opportunities it offers, had been developed. This allowed the group

members to take a less competitive approach to the exercise. Decisions about working with one another to reach a common goal, agreeing to follow or lead one another, without being competitive, now were considered.

Diana Halperin (2001) described the purposeful use of activity, with bilingual elders who were separated by language and cultural barriers, to find commonality and accept differences, take risks, and find a strengthened identity in the pursuit of shared goals (p. 27). A translator was used for the Spanish-speaking participants.

> The untested assumptions and biases of some of the members interfered with the group's work and with the building of a sense of commitment and shared goals.
>
> For the group to achieve its purpose, this problem had to be faced, relatively early in the beginning stage. The following excerpt describes the beginning of the process.
>
> An essential task for the worker was to address everyone's assumptions and biases about differences as they arose. Lorraine's humor and engagement expanded greatly in the group, and she became a strong group leader.
>
> Her initial feelings about language difference probably represented the most polarized end of the spectrum and an important one for the group to explore. In an early session in the group, the group and worker were addressing the need of the English speakers to remain quiet while information was translated into Spanish.

Lorraine: Well, I think that all of the Spanish speakers mostly understand English even though they can't speak it.

Worker: Ask them if that's true.

(Lorraine's comment is translated.)

(All the Spanish-speaking members shake their heads "no.")

Lorraine (looking shocked with her hand up by her mouth):
That never occurred to me. I always thought they understood . . .

Raising her consciousness about how the "other" group members experienced communication became the first step in Lorraine's (and the other English speakers') increased sensitivity toward the experience of her fellows.

The topic of understanding manifested itself week after week. The worker and the group kept challenging each other. "How do we make ourselves clear to each other in here?" "How will the audience understand all of us?" There was a great deal of exploring of body language through theatre and movement exercises. The dependence upon language lessened with the growth of other skills and levels of trust. (Halperin, pp. 39-40)

Claire Kaplan (2001) discusses arts-based activity groups that culminate with a performance. These groups have three purposes, ". . . all of which are important separately, but none of which can be achieved without the others. These three purposes are: (1) the skill-acquisition purposes, (2) the performance-based purpose, and (3) the socio-emotional purpose" (p. 48).

Kaplan commented on the interconnected, three-fold purpose and the unique challenges this presents to the worker. Kaplan's writing resonated with me and accurately described some of the challenges I experienced in the formation and implementation of the intergenerational singing group.

Ruth Middleman in her milestone book, *The Non-Verbal Method in Working with Groups* (1968, reissued in 1982), emphasized that the activity becomes the tool or vehicle that affects the intrapsychic and it has an effect on the interpersonal level. "I used the analogy of the times . . . program is a tool." She urged us to think of program more as putty than hammer, i.e., a tool that also changes as it is used (1982, p. 3).

Brandler and Roman (1999) wrote thoughtfully and comprehensively about the varied uses of activities. They said that often members in groups find:

> . . . it (is) possible to get what they needed from the group experience by talking with each other. Many clients we see, however, find this kind of communication impossible. They are unaccustomed to expressing deeply felt emotions directly . . . They struggle to clarify their thoughts and feel inadequate and self-conscious . . .
>
> Some populations find alternative ways of communicating feeling to be more natural and comfortable. Children, for example express themselves more naturally in play and fantasy. A foster children's group assignment to make a picture autobiography becomes a tool to address the terrible grief these youngsters feel

about the loss of family. Other groups may use music as a means of expression. Residents of a shelter for the homeless, people who are often unable to sustain social relationships, regain a sense of dignity, and belonging by participating in a band . . . (p. 138)

Activities can be used for one or more of the of the following reasons:

- To reach out to clients unable to express themselves verbally
- To teach specific coping skills
- To help clients feel competent, worthwhile, and–through mastery–spiritually, emotionally, and intellectually rejuvenated
- To distance from a threatening subject matter in order to be able to engage in problem-solving
- To learn to share and work cooperatively towards common goals
- To engage clients selectively around an area in which painful material creates resistance
- To help clients express socially unacceptable feelings in a socially accepted manner
- To help develop greater frustration tolerance
- To provide individuals with an opportunity to experience and test out new roles
- To use the activity as a way to create successful movement towards verbal communication
- To help in diagnosis, interpretation, and treatment

The 11points referred to above (1999, pp. 138-140, and also in the first edition of their book, 1991, pp. 128-130) are a brief summary of Brandler and Roman's discussion.

Purpose

The literature above emphasized the purposeful use of activities. Purpose is an essential concept in group work theory and in its practice. Purpose also is a dynamic and evolving concept. It can change as the group develops. "The group's determination of purpose is an evolutionary process" (Kurland and Salmon, 1998). It is generally accepted among group workers that "a group's purpose is defined as the ends that the groups will pursue collectively–what is anticipated that the groups and its members will achieve together" (Northen and Kurland, p. 175).

As purpose is the end, what is to be achieved, the content, what one actually does to achieve the group's purpose, is the means. All too often, content and purpose are confused. This frequently leaves members perplexed and disgruntled. They need to know why they are doing an activity; they need to know the reasons.

Clarity of purpose is crucial if the group is to be successful. The group members need to understand, participate in and "sign on" to the purpose of the group. When this occurs, it provides goals for the group, and often for the individual members, as well. Dominique Steinberg described it in this way: "Individual goals reflect those personal needs and desires that group members bring to the group, and group purpose is the common cause that ties those needs and desires together" (Steinberg, 1997).

When the stated purpose is unclear, deceptive or fuzzy, the ultimate result often is the failure of the group. Group members will stop coming if they feel that the group is not responsive to their needs and desires. Workers, therefore ". . . need to know in advance what they will say to the group about their vision for the group, their hopes for group accomplishments, and their reason for, and the agency's interest in, bringing the group members together" (Kurland and Salmon, 1998, p. 47).

THE PROCESS OF GROUP DEVELOPMENT

The CAPS program is designed to address the emotional needs of children who are having academic difficulties and are in danger of failing or dropping out or falling substantially behind at an early age. The children frequently are isolated from community support, live in poverty, and lack stable housing. A purposeful use of activities such as Tai-Chi, the use of visual arts, games of all kinds, and other activities are used to engage these students in the process of creating a cohesive group experience. The group environment nurtures the individual and the children learn from and support each other.

While working in my summer position at the Senior Residence, many of the seniors were eager to form relationships with me. Some engaged me in conversation about the uncertainties of their health. Others embraced my presence as an opportunity to share their life's experiences and their perceptions of what they can still accomplish. Many of these seniors live in isolation and some battle the feeling of solitude on a daily basis. Some seniors use the activities at the Center as an opportunity to connect with others of the community or other residents. One of their Center-based activities that was developed was a singing group–an open membership group–that met weekly. As is usual with open groups, there was a fluctuating membership. It consisted of about 15 people, free to participate or not, as they preferred. The group's leader, a social worker, was in the process of phasing out of her position due to funding problems. As my summer placement came to an end, many seniors expressed an interest in learning more about the program I coordinated in the school. The interest that the seniors expressed in establishing a relationship with the elementary school children, and thinking about the positive personal impact the two age groups might have on each other, led me to approach the Director of Social Services at the residence about the possibility of forming an intergenerational singing group. She was enthusiastic about the idea, and we entered the planning stage.

The Director, who is not a group worker, and I met several times to discuss group formation. We both recognized the "need" in both populations. Many of the participants live isolated from community life. Through the mutual aid process participants in both groups will problem-solve together and make decisions related to their singing and any issues that may develop. The Director and I also discussed the content and use of specific activity. We both agreed that the purpose of the activity was central in the group experience. I suggested that success in this joint endeavor was not in terms of something like: . . . "games won, ceramics produced, or information learned, but in what the experience meant to the participants" (Malekoff, 1997, p. 34). I felt that coming together on an agreed-upon task, which also provided pleasure, enjoyment, and a sense of competence, would serve as a counterforce to the isolation some in both age groups may experience in their daily lives.

We both agreed that although the groups would not rehearse together regularly, the groups would come together periodically to meet each other and sing together, and we would look to a late spring performance as an ending activity. We would suggest activities, such as correspondence and the exchange of art projects, that could act as vehicles to help establish relationships between the seniors and the children.

John, a social-work intern who had no training in group work, would be assigned to lead the senior group, along with a co-facilitator who had musical skill and ability in leading musical groups. He would work with both groups. The Director of the Social Services at the residence did not want the seniors to be informed about the possibility of correspondence between the groups. Her concern was that this would "scare the seniors off" from participating in the group. The lack of clarity and agreement about this caused difficulties later in the process of group formation.

There was agreement that the intergenerational group would have a dual purpose. One was related to learning the basics of singing/voice, and the second was related to a socio-emotional purpose which included building a sense of community. There were no pre-group interviews of the elders prior to the first meeting. Flyers were distributed in the residence to advertise the new singing group and recruit participants. However, the flyer did *not* specify that it was for an intergenerational singing group.

During this process, I introduced the idea of an intergenerational group to the children. Pre-group interviews were held to make an assessment of prospective group members and to prepare them for group entry. The purpose of the group was spelled out and individual expectations were made clear. A common concern among the students was that they could not sing, but they liked the idea of forming a relationship with a senior and approved the idea of becoming a group member. The group consisted of eight fifth-grade children, four girls, four boys, all aged 10- to 11-years-old.

Children's First Meeting

I used an icebreaker to start the first meeting with the children, so they could relax, as well as gain sureness about the names of all group members. An excerpt from the first session follows:

> *Worker: Thank you, everyone, for introducing yourselves. I would like us to talk a little more about the singing group.*
>
> *Salvatore: When are we going to meet the seniors?*
>
> *Worker: That's a very good question, Salvatore, and I will answer your question but first I'd like to begin by explaining to all of you the purpose of our meetings and how often we will meet, and lastly when we meet with the singing group of the senior residence.*
>
> *Jesus: Are we going to perform in a show?*
>
> *Gloria: What kind of song are we going to sing?*
>
> *Worker: Pablo, John, and I will meet to discuss the type of songs that we will practice. Also, I'd like to hear your thoughts and some suggestions.*

Salvatore: Can we suggest some rap songs? Or maybe some rhythm and blues?

Tannika: Seniors can't rap.

Worker: But we can decide as a group how to include songs you want to do. Remember that the purpose of this group is to learn some of the basics of voice and have fun. It is also a place where we will need to learn to respect each other's ideas, listen to each other and be willing to give and take constructive criticism. We are going to have the opportunity to talk about our own preconceived ideas of the elders in the senior singing group. Salvatore asked earlier if we are going to meet the seniors. We definitely will meet them at some point as the singing groups develop, but we also can begin by writing to them and exchanging some art projects. How does that sound to you?

Nora: Are we going to be assigned a senior, like a pen pal?

Worker: Yes, you will be assigned a senior. I can't promise they will all write back, but I am sure they will all be very interested in hearing about you and from you.

(At this point everyone begins to talk at the same time with a great deal of excitement.)

Worker: I can see that all of you are very excited, but I'd like to answer Jesus's question. We will be performing at the senior residence during the spring so it's very important that we work together and remain focused.

First Meeting with the Senior Singing Group

Seventeen seniors came to a meeting in response to the flyer, including some members of the previous singing group that had been established. John introduced himself as the worker, and Pablo who will accompany the group with the guitar and lead the rehearsals.

John asked everyone to introduce themselves and explained the purpose of the group as coming together to sing and to possibly establish a correspondence with a singing group in an elementary school. The majority of the seniors immediately expressed concern because they felt that this was not only singing but there was another agenda to the group. Some seniors expressed concern because of their difficulty in writing, and others just shook their heads in disagreement. Pablo proceeded to introduce the first song for practice. It was a song of the Beatles, "There Is a Place." Several seniors expressed their feeling about having to sing songs to which they cannot relate. Grudgingly, they proceeded to practice. However, they enjoyed the singing and Pablo's musical leadership. Many returned weekly to sing together. Some dropped out, and since it was an open group, new members were welcomed whenever they came. Bill, one of the most active members of the residence, played a leadership role.

After a month of group meetings and singing I met with the Director again regarding the idea of revisiting the purpose of the activity with the senior group. I felt many program opportunities for establishing strong relationships between the age groups were missed. The dual purpose was not established and that had a limiting quality as a result. The Director was reluctant to discuss this with the group.

Intergenerational Singing Group–First Meeting

The two groups met for the first time about six weeks after they started to rehearse. Art projects were presented to the seniors, who were pleased to receive them and meet the children. There was much good feeling. The children were particularly drawn to Bill, who was very positive and energetic in his response to the children. They bonded quickly. Another senior, Camille, joined the children in active dancing because "the young ones made me feel young again." The joint meeting lacked structure and organization, but it made the process real to both age groups and it provided a promising foundation for future meetings.

About a week later, Bill died suddenly and unexpectedly. The children were moved and upset and quickly planned a good-bye-mourning ritual. One of the children wrote a poem which they recited together and released helium balloons to commemorate his life and his importance to them, although they met only once.

Sadness

Written by Nora

Dedicated to Bill

Gloria: When we heard the news
That you had passed away
Our hearts were broken into little pieces.

Chorus: R.I.P. Rest in Peace
R.I.P. Rest in Peace

Tannika: Please remember that you are in our hearts
We'll be there by the Hudson River
Praying to God to bring you back.

Chorus: R.I.P. Rest in Peace (twice)

Manny: We know it was the first time we saw you
But the best one of all
We didn't think it was the last
Until you passed away.

Chorus: R.I.P. Rest in Peace (twice)

Gloria: Tears came running down our face
Happy frowns turned upside down
Then we decided to get balloons
Write messages to show we LOVE you.

Chorus: R.I.P. Rest in Peace (4 times)

Everyone: We just want you to know that we love you BILL!

Intergenerational Singing Group–Second Meeting

Prior to the second meeting of the intergenerational singing group, John, the student intern, and I had several planning meetings. The children and the seniors had been paired for the first joint meeting, and to the extent possible, that arrangement was to be continued. The format for the meeting was established.

We wanted the seniors and the children to have the opportunity to talk with one another. The children were in a closed group. Membership was stable. The seniors were in an open group, and membership was expected to change. I discussed in advance of the joint meeting the fact that some elders who were at the first meeting might not be at the second because they had a doctor's appointment or may not be feeling well. The children were surprised and puzzled over the fact that daily activities often revolved around how the elders felt physically, or medical appointments.

I opened the discussion with the intergenerational group by talking briefly about the purpose of bringing them together–in terms of the potential for relationships and the fun of singing together, as well. The children were invited to talk about their experience. Some of the children talked about how surprised they were that the elders "had the lungs to sing loud."

Some of the children said they expected the seniors to be cranky people who disliked children, but instead they found them to be funny, and kind, and loving. The elders also voiced their thoughts. One said that she doesn't generally like to be around children, but this experience was very special to her. She enjoyed the children's company and their energy.

Bill's death was discussed and several of the seniors talked about how much Bill enjoyed being with the children. The children talked about the emotional experience of sending off helium-filled balloons from the school yard with messages to Bill attached and how pleased they had been to know him. To be able to talk about an older adult who had been important to them, and express feelings of loss and caring, and to be heard, was a powerful experience for them.

Each group performed for the other. The youngsters did a rap version of "If I Was a Rich Man," which the elders enjoyed immensely. The elders sang a Beatles song, "Imagine" for the children and then they sang several songs for the first time together that they had both rehearsed in their own age groups. There were refreshments and conversation at the end, and the experience for both age groups and the staff was gratifying and meaningful.

Intergenerational Singing Group–Third Meeting

The third meeting of the intergenerational group was to be the final meeting, and it was to be a performance for the residents of the Senior Residence. "Endings with groups are particularly complicated because they occur on three levels: the relationship between group members and the worker is coming to an end, the relationships among the group members are ending, and the group as an entity is concluded and will cease to exist. The worker needs to be cognizant simultaneously of the multiple meanings on all three levels" (Kurland and Salmon, 1998, p.132).

This was even more complicated for the children because the worker would be leaving the agency as the grant funding the CAPS program was coming to an end. A long-term, meaningful relationship between the worker and the children would be ending.

Common reactions to this stage of the group's life include denial, regression and flight. With the children, it was regression, as shown by a great deal of confrontation and conflict among them. Pablo, the guitar player said, . . . "These last few group meetings felt just like when we first started." I led several discussions with the youngsters about termination, how much I valued the group and them, and how much the elders enjoyed working with them. Essentially their destructive behavior was interrupted. I was able through the use of reminiscence and evaluation to help them move toward a more appropriate ending. The children talked about how challenged they felt by the program, and how good it was to perform for the elders and also, with just their own group, for their classmates. Some of the children wanted to continue a relationship with a senior.

The ending meetings with the seniors were led by the student intern. I was not present. An announcement was made telling them of the performance at the Senior Residence, but it appeared that there was little, if any, discussion. Some of the seniors said they were not ready to perform before an audience.

When it was time for the performance, all the children were present, but only half of the seniors appeared. Flight as a reaction was evident with the other elders. It appeared that they were, by their actions, dealing with the situation by saying, "I will leave this group before you leave me."

The children were disappointed about that, as were the seniors who were there, but the performance went on. It was enjoyed thoroughly by the audience and the participants, and this positive reception was strong affirmation for the entire experience. The children had developed more positive social skills, and they appeared more confident, more enthusiastic, and appreciative of older people as well. The seniors who participated had an experience of joining a mixed age group, and singing and interacting with younger people. Stereotypes were challenged and the joy of activity was experienced. The seniors, in discussion, described it as a renewing of life.

REFLECTIONS

Group work is, and has been, a way of work that is useful and significant in meeting the needs of many seniors and children. I was fortunate to work for a settlement house where group work was valued, endorsed, and practiced. However, although there was a philosophical support for the theory and way of work, there was a lack of workers prepared educationally in this method of social work practice. This factor had an effect on the success of the intergenerational singing group discussed in this paper. "To be a group worker today is to be lonely" (Kurland and Salmon, 2002). Emily Wolff Newman described it this way:

> It is very isolating to be a social group worker today. Social group work is a method of practice that seems to be a whisper if at all audible in most graduate school programs. As result, there are few people trained in social work, and those of us who are, are the odd birds of our agencies. We are rarely surrounded by colleagues who share a similar group work philosophy or understanding. (Newman, 2000, p. 22)

Sharing group work literature while working on the intergenerational singing group with my colleagues was useful to them. Weekly planning meetings were initiated part way through the program and were helpful in the work with the seniors and children. All involved staff were given a showing of the film, "Close Harmony," and this was helpful in envisioning the power of the work in challenging stereotypes, building competence, and in bringing age groups together. The seniors and children benefited considerably in terms of relationships formed, and in feeling less isolated and more involved in a community. They also experienced the joy of singing together, and in learning new skills. Both groups felt challenged, and the children, in particular, felt they had met these challenges successfully. Group work with these age groups was the way to achieve these important benefits to two groups in great need. While much success was achieved in the process, more might have occurred with the elders if more of the professional staff were educated in group work practice and had the training to practice it. However, that was not the situation and despite it, the groups were largely successful.

Schools of social work slowly are bringing some group work courses back to the curriculum, as the power of purposeful activities is demonstrated again and again. As the process evolves, we have to be missionaries (as well as practitioners) for the method. It is a worthy calling.

NOTE

1. The "I" refers to Miriam Cusicanqui, Coordinator for the CAPS Program when this article was written.

REFERENCES

Aday, R.H., Sims, C.R., McDuffie, W., and Evans, E. (1996). Changing Children's Attitudes toward the Elderly: The Longitudinal Effects of an Intergenerational Partners Program. *Journal of Research in Childhood Education,* Vol. 10, pp. 143-151.

Brandler, S., and Roman, C. P. (1999). *Group Work: Skills and Strategies for Effective Interventions,* 2nd Edition. New York: The Haworth Press, Inc.

Burke, J. (1981). Young Children's Attitudes and Perceptions of Older Adults. *International Journal of Aging and Human Development,* Vol. 14, pp. 205-222.

Coyle, G. (1947). Group Work as a Method in Recreation. *In Group Experience and Democratic Values* (pp. 69-80). New York: The Woman's Press.

Dinolfo, D. (2004). Movement and Group Work (Unpublished paper). New York.

Halperin, D. (2001). The Play's the Thing: How Social Group Work and Theater Transformed a Group into a Community. *Social Work with Groups,* Vol. 24 (2) pp. 27-46.

Hummert, M.L. (1993). Age and Typicality of Judgments of Stereotypes of the Elderly: Perceptions of Elderly vs. Young Adults. *International Journal of Aging and Human Development,* Vol. 37, pp. 217-226.

Kaplan, C. (2001). The Purposeful Use of Performance in Groups: A New Look at the Balance of Task and Process. *Social Work with Groups,* Vol. 24(2), pp. 47-68.

Kurland, R., and Salmon, R. (1998). *Teaching a Methods Course in Social Work with Groups.* Alexandria, VA: Council on Social Work Education.

Kurland, R., and Salmon, R. (1998). Purpose: A Misunderstood and Misused Keystone of Group Work Practice. *Social Work with Groups,* Vol. 21(3), pp. 5-17.

Kurland, R., and Salmon, R. (In Press). Caught in the Doorway between Education and Practice: Group Work's Battle for Survival. In C. Cohen, M. Phillips, and M. Hansen (Eds.), *Think Group. Strength and Diversity in Group Work.* New York: The Haworth Press, Inc.

Malekoff, A. (1997). *Group Work with Adolescents: Principles and Practice.* New York: Guilford Press.

Mattaini, M., Lowery, C., and Meyer, C. (1998). *The Foundations of Social Work Practice.* Washington, DC: NASW Press.

Middleman, R. (1968). *The Non-verbal Method in Working with Groups.* New York: Association Press. Republished in 1982, Hebron, CT: Practitioners Press.

Newman, E.W. (2000). Pearls in the Muck. *Social Work with Groups,* Vol. 23(3), pp. 19-36.

Noble, N., Producer and Director (1981). *Close Harmony.* Oscar Winner, Best Short Documentary, 1981, Emmy Award, 1982. Washington, DC: National Council on Aging.

Northen, H., and Kurland, R. (2001). *Social Work with Groups.* New York: Columbia University Press.

Palmore, E. (1990). A*geism: Negative and Positive.* New York: Springer.

Pinquart, M., Wenzel, S., and Sorensen, S. (2000). Changes in Attitudes among Children and the Elderly Adults in Intergenerational Group Work. *Educational Gerontology,* Vol. 26(6), pp. 523-540.

Schnekenburger, E. (1995). Waking the Heart Up: A Writing Group's Story. *Social Work with Groups,* Vol. 18(4), pp. 19-40.

Shulman, L. (1971). Program in Group Work: Another Look. In William Schwartz and Serapio Zalba (Eds.), *The Practice of Group Work* (pp. 221-240). New York: Columbia University Press.

Steinberg, D. (1997). *The Mutual-Aid Approach to Working with Groups: Helping People Help Each Other.* Northvale, NJ: Jason Aronson, Inc.

Trecker, H. (1955). *Group Work: Foundations and Frontiers.* New York: Whiteside and William Morrow.

Vinter, R. (1974). Program Activities: An Analysis of Their Effects on Participant Behavior. In M. Sundel, P. Glasser, R. Sarri, and R. Vinter (Eds.), *Individual Change through Small Groups* (2nd ed., pp. 233-243). New York: Free Press.

Ward, C.R., Kemp, L.L., and Newman, S. (1996). The Effects of Participation in an Intergenerational Program on the Behavior of Residents with Dementia. *Activities, Adaptation, & Aging,* Vol. 20 (4), pp. 61-76.

Wilson, G., and Ryland, G. (1949). *Social Group Work Practice.* Boston: Houghton-Mifflin.

Wright, W. (1999). The Use of Purpose in On-going Activity Groups: A Framework for Maximizing the Therapeutic Impact. *Social Work with Groups,* Vol. 22(2/3), pp. 31-54.

Using the End of Groups
as an Intervention at End-of-Life

Ann Goelitz, MSW, CSW

SUMMARY. Support groups are an effective therapy at end-of-life. Patients with life-threatening illness and caregivers of the terminally ill have benefited from the mutual aid process provided by groups. Mutual aid is fostered by talking about feelings and developing group cohesion. Difficulty discussing the multiple issues of loss faced at end-of-life, including death and dying, can stifle sharing and impede this process. Group endings offer a unique opportunity to symbolically introduce these topics. This article explores the utilization of the group developmental stage of termination when facilitating groups for this population. *[Article copies available for a fee from The Haworth Document Delivery Service: 1-800-HAWORTH. E-mail address: <docdelivery@haworthpress.com> Website: <http://www. HaworthPress.com> © 2004 by The Haworth Press, Inc. All rights reserved.]*

KEYWORDS. End-of-life, support groups, developmental stages, termination, group cohesion, mutual aid

[Haworth co-indexing entry note]: "Using the End of Groups as an Intervention at End-of-Life." Goelitz, Ann. Co-published simultaneously in *Journal of Gerontological Social Work* (The Haworth Social Work Practice Press, an imprint of The Haworth Press, Inc.) Vol. 44, No. 1/2, 2004, pp. 211-221; and: *Group Work and Aging: Issues in Practice, Research, and Education* (ed: Robert Salmon, and Roberta Graziano) The Haworth Social Work Practice Press, an imprint of The Haworth Press, Inc., 2004, pp. 211-221. Single or multiple copies of this article are available for a fee from The Haworth Document Delivery Service [1-800-HAWORTH, 9:00 a.m. - 5:00 p.m. (EST). E-mail address: docdelivery@haworthpress.com].

INTRODUCTION

This article will explore the use of support groups at end-of-life. Specifically, the termination stage of groups will be examined as a means of symbolically addressing the multiple issues of loss encountered at this time of life. As the population ages and more and more individuals find themselves facing the possibility of imminent death, science continues to increase life expectancy so that end-of-life is also extended. Statistics compiled by the Centers for Disease Control reveal that in America deaths have reached an all time low at the same time as life expectancy has reached a high of 77.2 years (U.S. Department of Health and Human Services, 2003). These facts make it clear that psychosocially treating the terminally ill and their caregivers is a significant endeavor that warrants investigation.

Patients with incurable disease know that death may come at any time. Caregivers, who also live with this awareness, are constantly reminded of the vulnerability of life and of their own mortality. This can not only create a need for emotional support but also bring about isolation, depression, and anxiety. Many patients never receive help and/or can have difficulty discussing the losses that accompany illness. These losses include the patient's physical metamorphosis, lifestyle changes, effects on interpersonal relationships, loss of control, and anticipatory grief (Goelitz, 2001a & b).

Psychosocial care at end-of-life can help patients and caregivers cope with their loss. Research shows the influence of end-of-life care on depression, sleep patterns, mood, emotional well-being, and quality of life (QOL). QOL in particular has been improved by psychological interventions (Greer, 2002).

It is well-documented that support groups are an effective intervention at end-of-life. Groups can help by increasing psychological, social, and physiological well-being as they reduce isolation and encourage sharing of feelings related to illness and death. Through the mutual aid engendered by groups, individuals at end-of-life have the opportunity to obtain social support, express their emotions, and discuss issues of death and dying (Hardy and Riffle, 1993; Goelitz, 2001a; Goelitz, 2003; Gore-Felton and Spiegel, 1999).

To be successful, support groups at end-of-life need to develop cohesion, mutual aid, and intimacy as members share feelings and discuss topics of importance to them (Northen, 1988; Schwartz, 1971). Gore-Felton and Spiegel (1999) purport that introducing topics related to death and dying, and discussing associated feelings, can reduce anxiety, counter isolation, and help individuals at end-of-life regain a sense of control. They identify detoxifying dying as an essential ingredient of effective group therapy for patients with terminal illness.

The literature reveals that introducing and/or pursuing discussions related to these topics can be difficult for both group leaders and members. These topics are often not brought up as members utilize defense mechanisms to avoid them (Brown, 1991) and leaders collaborate, as one study finds, to the point of not even discussing the death of a group member (Gabriel, 1981; Hyland et al., 1984). This article will focus on how the group developmental stage of termination can be utilized as a vehicle for these types of discussions.

GROUP STAGE THEORY

The literature discusses the progression of support groups through developmental stages as members engage and their relationship with the group matures. Authors identify stages in various ways but all seem to agree that the stage of the group affects its dynamics and that awareness of stage theory can enable leaders to effectively assess group functionality. This can allow for optimal selection of group content and interventions (Kurland and Salmon, 1998; Northen, 1988).

Stage theory outlines group processes as beginning with planning and ending with termination. Kurland and Salmon (1998) describe four developmental stages: planning, beginning, middle, and ending. They attach certain characteristics and themes to each stage that relate to the growth needs of the group. For instance, beginnings and endings require more structure and active leadership to hold group members and provide stability as they navigate the transitions.

The termination stage of groups is a time of separation and the end of the group process. It is complicated because it involves not just the group ending, but also the severing of the members to leader relationship and of the relationship between the members (Kurland and Salmon, 1998). This is an important stage in that it can provide the opportunity to integrate and apply benefits gained from the group as the group experience is related to everyday life. If managed in this way by the leader, it can also help members to deal with old issues related to loss and separation (Northen and Kurland, 2001).

Members react to this stage with anger, denial, regression, and flight. Attendance can fall off as members start to disengage; criticisms of the group, the leader, or other members may be expressed; members can be clingy, asking why the group has to end, or may become detached and removed. Kacen (1999) found that anxiety levels increased for members at this phase of groups. Leaders can also have their own reactions to endings. For example, they may rush to introduce new material in an unconscious effort to prolong the group or to add to its validity. Members can also have this tendency (Kurland and Salmon, 1998; Northen, 1988).

Group leaders can help members through this phase by providing linkages to alternate means of support and by encouraging evaluation, recapitulation, and review (Whittaker, 1970). Articulation of feelings related to endings is important. This can be accomplished via reminiscence and can be encouraged by the group leader. Reminding members of the forthcoming separation can also aid members and allow the termination process to occur more naturally (Kurland and Salmon, 1998).

END OF GROUPS AT END-OF-LIFE

End-of-life groups tend to focus on physical symptoms, medical treatment, and information sharing (Goelitz, 2001a). This can limit intimacy as no real feelings are exchanged. Brown (1991) discusses the importance of members engaging in resolving emotional issues by sharing feelings in order to increase understanding and promote change. Group cohesiveness and mutual aid require intimacy in order to develop (Schwartz, 1971).

Using the group ending as a means to introduce the topics of death and dying in end-of-life groups can help to facilitate discussion of associated feelings. Not only will this improve group functioning as it increases intimacy, cohesion and mutual aid but it will allow members to get the support they need, reducing isolation and creating a space for them to integrate their experience, resolve conflicts, increase understanding, and regain hope (Goelitz, 2001a).

Most end-of-life support groups are time-limited, meeting weekly for a specified period of time ranging from six to ten sessions. This format gives leaders the chance to bring up termination during orientation as they let members know how long the group will last and throughout the group as they remind them of the number of sessions remaining.

In a series of caregiver support groups, facilitated by the author, with family members caring for the terminally ill, the group ending was introduced as a topic halfway through, in the fifth session. Group members generally tried to ignore the topic or at times even got angry at the leader for bringing it up so soon when, as they said, things were just getting started. According to the theories of Garland, Jones, and Kolodny (1973), this reflects their attempts to avoid or forestall terminating. By the sixth session, after repeated attempts, they were able to talk about it directly, and by the eighth, to relate it to other endings in their lives.

CASE EXAMPLES

In the sixth session of one group, the author reminded members of the group ending and asked them if they would like to do anything special to mark the occasion. Their ambivalence was expressed through their suggestions. Wanting to continue the group, to meet physically (this was a telephone group), or to communicate via e-mail after it ended suggested denial of the ending and an attempt to stop it from happening. The announcement that "the group had brought up a lot of feelings" which caused one member to start individual therapy indicated her beginning to detach from the group. In the next session, members complained that the ending seemed too soon and was happening before they were very connected, at the same time as they commented on liking the stories shared in the group because they helped get them in touch with feelings. This led to a discussion of the difficulties of caring for the dying:

Judy: Seems too soon for the group to end . . .

Susan: We still have time, don't we?

Facilitator: After this session we have three more so we are getting close to the end.

Judy: We're not so connected yet. People have missed sessions and it's harder on the phone.

Facilitator: Does it make it difficult to think about ending when you aren't even connected yet?

Sally: I wish we could have a regular group where we could see each other. I do like the stories though. They get me in touch with my feelings.

Mary: Does anyone know about case managers? I would like someone to do some of what they do.

Susan: I don't think all case managers do the same thing. Sometimes they can help provide facts and the process of fact finding helps with making decisions. We have to be able to delegate to get our jobs done.

Facilitator: Is that the kind of story that you like to hear, Sally–other people's experiences with caregiving?

Sally: I like learning from everyone's experiences and I like the sharing of feelings. Mother will only die once. Life is changing. I want to know about the feelings.

Facilitator: There's so much loss in caring for a sick loved one, and so many endings. It's not just the group ending you are dealing with but all kinds of endings.

Judy: I hate to say this but I'm jealous of Joyce (another group member whose father had died recently). It's so hard to see my mother-in-law.

Mary: It (death) would be a relief. This thing is always with you. Not that you don't care but when see that it could go on for a long time, it's only human . . .

Judy: If my mother-in-law knew how she was (she had Alzheimer's disease and was not aware), she would not want to be fed.

Mary: Sometimes my son is unresponsive and sometimes he recognizes me. Either way, I feel as though my care is a way of honoring him.

Facilitator: So you're left with feeling both the desire to honor and the wish for it to end–it's tough to have both feelings.

In the next and eighth session, the leader talked about how the group ending when they were not even connected yet was like the possibility of their loved ones dying too soon, using the group ending to again introduce the topic of death and dying. This caused members to talk about the group ending and ways they could mark the occasion, moving away from the difficult discussion of death to the more palatable idea of the group terminating. Members expressed their anger and frustration as they talked about problems they saw with the group–inconsistent attendance, despite the commitment they had all made, causing the group to be incomplete when members were absent which also changed the group chemistry; difficulties connecting in the group; and not liking the silence when no one talked. They also talked about how they could bare their souls and even say things they might not be proud of. Finally, after exhausting these topics, which also expressed a myriad of feelings reflecting the loss in their lives, they were able to talk about difficult decisions related to their loved one's imminent death and articulate related feelings of fear, sadness, and loss of control:

Susan: Silence is difficult on the phone. We can't see facial expressions so don't know what it means.

Facilitator: Just like your loved one's silence is difficult.

Mary: We're bringing Brad (her sick son) home. I'm nervous but I want to try again. I think it would help to have a case manager.

Judy: You might want to try to look for warning signs for when it's too much for you. We always try to do too much.

Facilitator: Setting limits and finding boundaries that work for you is important and can help you feel less out of control. There is so much loss of control when caring for someone who is sick.

Mary: And there's always a crisis. Hard to make decisions when in crisis. I'll try to think things through and discuss with my husband. We'll also have two shifts of help so I can be with my family in the evening.

Sally: Mother seems to feel safe in the nursing home but she is talking about going home at some point in the future.

Facilitator: You sound confused about that.

Sally: Well, I don't understand. I think she's better off in the nursing home where she feels safe. I try to talk to her about it but she doesn't respond and just says she wants to go home.

Tracy: No response is so hard.

Sally: I would almost prefer a negative response.

Group members: Don't say that. A negative response is much worse. It's better to have no response than a negative response.

Facilitator: You have enough negativity–losing your loved one as you knew them and your way of life. It's scary to listen to their negative thoughts as well.

Program activities can help prepare members for group endings (Toseland, 1995). The last session of these groups was always composed of activities designed by group members. These included sharing stories about their loved ones such as what they were like before they got sick; telling what they liked and would take from the group; and sharing hope, pledges, and plans for when the group ended. These activities allowed for evaluation, recapitulation, and review of both the group and the end-of-life process.

Some particularly poignant comments came out of the last session of one group where members had decided to share stories about loved one, experiences as a caregiver, and what they liked and would take from the group:

Sally: It isn't easy to get out of being alive. A friend of mine told me that and it is so true. I fear the process, not death and dying.

Facilitator: Do you want to say anything about the group?

Tracy: Support groups help. I'm more at ease. I've found comfort, not so alone knowing there are others out there doing the same thing, building that house. Talking releases fears and anxieties. I get ideas from the group. Glad I did it. Would like a reunion later (pause). I think very dearly of my mother and I don't want to lose her (she was crying as she said this).

Kathy: Group gives you strength, interesting to find out that you're not alone. Makes you stretch and grow. I'm surprised at what I say–I didn't realize what I was feeling. You get awareness. Wish you could meet my husband. Super human being. Thirty-six years of marriage . . .

(long silence)

Facilitator: Sally, did you want to share about the group?

Sally: Biggest thing put in touch with more feelings than thought I had and realized how much love this person (her mother). Made me go into therapy. Real surprise, I never had positive feelings about psychotherapy.

Facilitator: Anything else you want to share about your mother?

Sally: She has a touch of second childhood and is completely refusing to face her terminal illness.

(silence)

Mary: Susan said "Help me walk the path with grace and to see what good can come out of it." That helped me–it's a good approach. Sometimes may be overwhelmed but will just try to do the best. I liked having someone to talk to. We don't know each other and it's on the phone so I could say more. We won't cross paths again. It was comfortable and I could say more. Brad (her son) is two different people–one before the accident and one after. Can only get through this because of faith. Something special about him now. He's pure. People miss him even though he doesn't inter-act much. All the trappings of society are stripped away. Pleasure to be with him when he's not sick or having problems. When you're not looking, he steals your heart.

The comments about their loved ones were particularly touching since there had been so much anger toward them shared in the group. This is not uncommon since caregiving is a difficult and frequently thankless task performed for family members who are not at their best. The group ended with one member sharing a poem that expressed what many of them seemed to be saying in that last group session. The poem she chose was by Emily Dickinson (1961, p. 116):

> "Hope" is the thing with feathers–
> That perches in the soul–

CONCLUSION

The literature and case material demonstrate ways in which group endings offer a unique opportunity to symbolically introduce topics normally difficult to discuss. Through group discussions, feelings often held inside are aired. Death and dying detoxify as the fear of it loses some power. Members begin to feel less alone and develop understanding and hope.

This may be more valuable than we think. A recent *New York Times* article on old age reported how the elderly can fear and avoid all kinds of endings. They may find it harder to get off the phone, missing or ignoring the cues of conversations ending; or have difficulty finishing a book, taking longer than usual to read it. The article concluded by saying that it is better to face the ending than to avoid it because, "The longer you put something off, . . . the harder it is to face" (Dominus, February 22, 2004, Retrieved February 23, 2004 from *http://www. nytimes.com*). Toseland (1995) presents another point of view stating that older group members might actually tolerate group endings better than younger adults. He encourages helping members identify the positive aspects of the end of groups.

We as practitioners can facilitate this process. One way of doing this is by helping individuals at end-of-life talk about death and dying even when we have difficulty ourselves. Group endings can be a vehicle for these discussions, making the process easier and providing for a rich and rewarding group experience. This requires discussing termination early in the group process, reintroducing the topic as members resist and pull away from it, and relating group endings to the many losses experienced at end-of-life. These include lifestyle and relationship losses, as well as loss of control and the impending loss of life. The growing number of elderly individuals facing end-of-life issues makes this an important endeavor that has the potential to change many lives and to facilitate the process of death and dying.

REFERENCES

Brown, L. (1991). *Groups for Growth and Change*. White Plains, NY: Longman.

Dickinson, E. (1961). "Hope" is the thing with feathers. In Johnson, T. (Ed.), *The Complete Poems of Emily Dickinson*, Paperback Edition. Boston: Little, Brown, and Company.

Dominus, S. (February 22, 2004). Life in the Age of Old, Old Age. Retrieved February 23, 2004 from *http://www.nytimes.com*

Gabriel, M. (1991). Group therapists' countertransference reactions to multiple deaths from AIDS. *Clinical Social Work Journal*, 19(3), 279-291.

Garland, J., Jones, H., and Kolodny, R. (1973). A model for stages of development in social work groups. In Berstein, S. (Ed.), *Explorations in Group Work*. Boston: Milford House, Inc.

Goelitz, A. (2001). Dreaming their way into life: A group experience with oncology patients. *Social Work with Groups*, 24(1), 53-67.

Goelitz, A. (2001). Nurturing life with dreams: Therapeutic dream work with cancer patients. *Clinical Social Work Journal*, 29(4), 375-385.

Goelitz, A. (2003). When accessibility is an issue: Telephone support groups for caregivers. *Smith College Studies in Social Work*, 73(3), 385-394.

Gore-Felton, C., and Spiegel, D. (1999). Enhancing women's lives: The role of support groups among breast cancer patients. *Journal for Specialists in Group Work*, 24(3), 274-287.

Greer, S. (2002). Psychological intervention. The gap between research and practice. *Acta Oncology*, 41(3), 238-243.

Hardy, V., and Riffle, K. (1993). Support for caregivers of dependent elderly. *Geriatric Nursing*, 14(3), 161-164.

Hyland, J., Pruyser, H., Novotny, E., and Coyne, L. (1984). The impact of the death of a group member in a group of breast cancer patients. *International Journal of Group Psychotherapy*, 34(4), 617-626.

Kacen, L. (1999). Anxiety levels, group characteristics, and members' behavior in the termination stage of support groups for patients recovering from heart attacks. *Research on Social Work Practice*, 9(6), 656-672.

Kurland, R., and Salmon, R. (1998). *Teaching a Methods Course in Social Work with Groups*. Alexandria, VA: Council on Social Work Education.

Northen, H. (1988). *Social Work with Groups* (2nd ed.). New York: Columbia University Press.

Northen, H., and Kurland, R. (2001). *Social Work with Groups* (3rd ed.). New York: Columbia University Press.

Schwartz, W. (1971). Introduction: On the use of groups in social work practice. In Schwartz, W., and Zalba, S. (Eds.), *The Practice of Group Work*. New York: Columbia University Press.

Toseland, R. (1995). *Group Work with the Elderly and Family Caregivers*. New York: Springer Publishing Company.

U.S. Department of Health and Human Services (2003). HHS Study Finds Life Expectancy in the U.S. Rose to 77.2 Years in 2001. Retrieved October 6, 2003 from *http://www.merck.com/mrkshared/mmanual_home/sec1/4.jsp*

Whittaker, J. (1970). Models of group development: Implications for social group work practice. *Social Service Review*, 44(3), 308-322.

Group Field Instruction:
A Model
for Supervising Graduate Students
Providing Services to Older People

Barbara H. Rinehart, PhD
Roberta Graziano, DSW

SUMMARY. In order to meet the need for a qualified and professionally-educated work force to assist the increasing number of individuals
living into advanced years, a work-study Master of Social Work program that utilizes a unique group model of Field Supervision as part of a
specially designed gerontology curriculum was developed. This article
describes the program, the effect of the group Field Supervision model
on students, who were experienced employees already working with
older adults and their families, and the outcomes. The enhanced level of
knowledge and skill gained by the students was of substantial benefit to
their elderly clients. *[Article copies available for a fee from The Haworth Document Delivery Service: 1-800-HAWORTH. E-mail address: <docdelivery@
haworthpress.com> Website: <http://www.HaworthPress.com> © 2004 by The
Haworth Press, Inc. All rights reserved.]*

KEYWORDS. Group field instruction, older adults, a master's degree
work-study program, group work

[Haworth co-indexing entry note]: "Group Field Instruction: A Model for Supervising Graduate Students
Providing Services to Older People." Rinehart, Barbara H., and Roberta Graziano. Co-published simultaneously in *Journal of Gerontological Social Work* (The Haworth Social Work Practice Press, an imprint of
The Haworth Press, Inc.) Vol. 44, No. 1/2, 2004, pp. 223-242; and: *Group Work and Aging: Issues in Prac-
tice, Research, and Education* (ed: Robert Salmon, and Roberta Graziano) The Haworth Social Work Practice
Press, an imprint of The Haworth Press, Inc., 2004, pp. 223-242. Single or multiple copies of this article are
available for a fee from The Haworth Document Delivery Service [1-800-HAWORTH, 9:00 a.m. - 5:00 p.m.
(EST). E-mail address: docdelivery@haworthpress.com].

http://www.haworthpress.com/web/JGSW
© 2004 by The Haworth Press, Inc. All rights reserved.
Digital Object Identifier: 10.1300/J083v44n01_13

Increasing numbers of individuals in our society living into advanced years have underscored the need for a qualified and professionally educated work force to assist them. Graduate schools of social work are developing various educational models to recruit students who will be able to respond to the wide range of needs of this increasingly diverse and often frail aging population. The Hunter College School of Social Work, which pioneered in the development of a work-study program more than 30 years ago (Salmon and Walker, 1981), had not addressed the need for workers to practice in this growing field of gerontology until recently. This article describes a program that utilizes, as part of a specially designed gerontology curriculum, a unique group model of Field Supervision with students who are also experienced bachelor's-level workers in community agencies serving older adults in New York City.

BACKGROUND OF PROGRAM

The "Aging and Health" Work-Study MSW Program at the Hunter College School of Social Work, a grant-funded pilot project, was designed to address the significant and well-documented shortage of professionally-educated social workers who have expertise in meeting the social and health-related needs of older adults. At present, many workers serving seniors are lacking in professional training and tend to be deficient in the knowledge and skills necessary to properly address the complex issues of the elderly. Several educational initiatives have been under way–notably the collaborative effort between the John A. Hartford Foundation's "Strengthening Geriatric Social Work" program and the Council on Social Work Education's "SAGE–SW" (Strengthening Aging and Gerontology Education for Social Work) project. Gerontology concentrations have begun to be offered at some graduate schools of social work, but these efforts have centered primarily around generating interest in gerontology among full-time students in traditional two-year educational programs.

By contrast, the "Aging and Health" Program–*the first work-study social work graduate program in Aging and Health in the country*–admits bachelor-level agency workers with both experience and a commitment to working with older adults. This focus is consistent with the mission of the Hunter College School of Social Work–the only public school of social work in New York City–which is to educate social work professionals who will provide services to underserved and disadvantaged individuals, families, groups, and communities regardless of age, ethnicity, culture, religion, disability, or sexual orientation.

The School has a long history of preparing employees of social agencies for professional practice through its work-study program, the One Year Residency (OYR) Program (Haffey and Starr, 1988), which offers experienced workers the opportunity to earn the MSW degree in 2 1/2 years while continuing to work full-time. The "Aging and Health" Program, part of the OYR structure, provides: (1) tuition scholarships; (2) a course of study that includes in-depth classroom exposure to theory, policy, and practice issues affecting older adults, with a special interdisciplinary focus on health issues of the elderly within a multicultural urban environment; (3) a full-time Professional Development Counselor (PDC) who functions as a faculty advisor, mentor, and advocate; (4) a job-based internship or Field Practicum, designed to facilitate the learning and application of new skills; and (5) a full-time Field Instructor, based at the School of Social Work, to supervise the internship of the participating student, and provide group supervision.

The specific purpose of the Aging and Health Program is to educate the next generation of social work practitioners so that they are able to serve their older clients in the most effective way possible. The Professional Development Counselor position was included as a major component of the "Aging and Health" Program from the outset, but in order to achieve purpose, and to meet the special needs of the students and their agencies, more was required.

The Students

The students are full-time employees of agencies serving older adults in New York City. To date, there have been two cohorts of students–15 in the first class, 14 in the second–and a third cohort is being recruited now. The students are about equally divided between administrators and those in direct practice. They are ethnically diverse, including African-American, Caribbean-American (both French- and English-speaking), Latino/a (from at least six different countries), Chinese, Russian, Jewish-American, Irish-American, and Italian-American students. About half of the students are immigrants, some quite recent; a number of them received their undergraduate educations in countries outside the U.S., in a language other than English. Their ages range from late twenties to mid-fifties. Twenty-seven, or 90%, of the students are women, a proportion not unusual in social work. Many of the students are married and have family responsibilities; some are responsible for aging parents or other family members as well; a small number of the students have health problems or disabilities. All of the students must have completed at least two years of social work agency experience before applying to the program; some have worked for many more years.

The Agencies

The agencies that employ the students are located in four of New York City's boroughs. The majority of the program sites are in Brooklyn and Queens, the two most populous and most ethnically diverse boroughs. (Indeed, Queens is the most diverse county in the nation.) The programs represented all serve community-dwelling elders and include senior centers, senior housing, case management, elder abuse programs, adult day care, geriatric health clinics, geriatric substance abuse residences, and mental health clinics. Some are small free-standing agencies; others are satellite programs of large agencies with many sites.

SCHOOL-BASED FIELD INSTRUCTOR

Precursor of the Group Supervision Model

The group Field Supervision model that evolved out of the Aging and Health Program has strong ties to innovations created for past and current work-study scholarship programs at HCSSW. It has become clear over time that part-time students are more likely than full-time students to view both time and emotional demands as greater than expected (Potts, 1992); that programs of this type attract older students, many of them minority and women, with multiple family and personal demands on their time in addition to their work and school responsibilities; and that working full-time while in school seems to hinder the psychological adjustment of social work students. Thus, a built-in "support system" was called for, and the Professional Development Counselor (PDC) position was developed some 15 years ago (Salmon, Haffey, Blau, and Johnson, 1993) to meet that need and now is implemented in all grant-funded components of the OYR (work-study) program. The PDC was envisioned as a faculty advisor and professional mentor who is with–and for–the students throughout their time in the program, working primarily in a mutual-aid group (Graziano, Salmon, and Berman, 2002):

. . . the faculty advising role and the mutual aid engendered through group meetings were considered of critical importance to students, with the understanding that social work education exacts emotional, developmental, and learning demands not found in the traditional academic setting. The conflicting demands of education, work, and family life often were extremely difficult for the working student to manage. It was understood that the students' social network would have to become an important resource in the school environment, and that group meetings would serve as instruments of help and mutual aid.

Rationale for School-Based Field Instructor

In the process of planning an educational program for workers in community-based organizations providing services to older people and their families, the strong need for a school-based Field Instructor emerged. It was evident from the agency-based research conducted in the development phase of the Aging and Health Program that many of the community agencies either didn't have experienced MSWs to provide social work field supervision, or that such staff were already feeling overburdened by heavy work loads. Thus, when the proposal was put forth for the Aging and Health Program at HCSSW, a full-time school-based and funded Field Instructor was included.

Social work schools, in partnership with field work agencies, have experimented over the years with different approaches to field supervision (Marshack and Glassman, 1991). The predominant model of field work teaching is a one-on-one method of field instruction: one field practicum instructor, an employee of the field practice agency, to supervise one social work student. However, since the 15 students accepted into the first cohort of this program were placed in 14 different sites throughout Brooklyn and Queens (with one student placed in Manhattan), it became clear very quickly that one Field Instructor could not work with 15 students using the traditional one-on- one field instruction model. Other models of field instruction began to be explored. As stated by Marshack and Glassman (1991), ". . . student education requires a commitment operationalized through agency and school structure, and implemented by educators who are prepared to take risks" (p. 85).

The primary goals of the field practicum experience for the Aging and Health students were to maximize their learning as social work practitioners in the field of aging. The use of a small group, composed of students with similar interests, seemed to be an ideal way for them to learn about different types of aging settings, different types of practice, and individual aging issues. Students would have the opportunity to share their practice experiences, to raise questions, to support one another, and also to begin to challenge one another in a safe environment, through a process facilitated by a skilled Field Instructor. It would draw upon the theoretical underpinnings of group work practice, and group supervision (Shulman, 1993).

Group field instruction is not new. "Group field instruction can be used as a primary method of field instruction. Social work groups are known for their effectiveness as learning systems through their processes of mutual aid, consensual validation, and feedback" (Marshack and Glassman, 1991; also, see Abels, 1983; Getzel, Goldberg, and Salmon, 1971; and Getzel and Salmon, 1985). However, this model is still the exception to the rule, rather than a normal part of field education programs in graduate schools of social work. Thus, it was important that the Field Instructor be ". . . required to have knowledge in the areas of social work practice, educational methods, and group methods" (Marshack and Glassman, 1991, p. 89). In this particular program, the designated Field Instructor was a group worker with over 25 years of experience, both as clinician and as administrator, working in the field of aging in community-based agencies, similar to the work sites of the students in this program.

Agency-Based Task Supervisor

In the Aging and Health program, with its school-based Field Instructor, an on-site Task Supervisor was particularly important in order to foster and maintain a strong tie between the school and the agency. A Task Supervisor, an experienced social worker at each agency, was needed to oversee the work assignments of the student, and to help maintain the balance between "student" assignments and "worker" assignments. The Task Supervisor was available to respond to day-to-day questions, thus becoming an important link between the school-based Field Instructor and the student's field practicum work with older individuals.

GROUP FIELD INSTRUCTION MODEL

In group work, there are four important stages in the process: planning, beginnings, middles, and endings (Kurland and Salmon, 1998).

These four stages were used as a theoretical framework for the group model of Field Instruction developed for the Aging and Health program.

Planning Stage

Even before developing the group itself, and before the field practicum year actually began, the school faculty advisor (PDC) and the Field Instructor met with designated agency personnel, including the Task Supervisor, to plan for the field practicum year. The discussion included the use of a group work model for field instruction, appropriate assignments that would provide opportunities for experience in several minor practice methods, and emphasis on the need for the employer to reduce the student/employee's work load to accommodate the educational demands of the field practicum year. A written contract was then prepared by the PDC to confirm the plan for the fieldwork experience in aging practice. All persons involved reviewed and signed the contract.

Group Composition

Since moving from traditional one-on-one field education to a group model of supervision was going to be a new experience, with new demands and opportunities, it was important to make the group compatible and small enough to make it workable. Fortunately, both cohorts of Aging and Health students were divided between direct practice and administration (7-8 casework or group work students and 7-8 administration students). Thus, the field practicum supervisory sessions–which were called "seminars"–were divided into two groups–one casework/group work seminar and one administration seminar.

Meeting Place and Time

Determining a place and time to meet was particularly difficult for the first cohort of students. Scheduling was the most challenging part of implementing this group work model of field instruction. Students in the OYR Program at HCSSW come to school one day a week during their field placement year. They carry a full load of academic classes during this academic year. Once or twice, meetings were held during students' lunch hour, but that was difficult since this was the only time they had to catch a breath, socialize, follow-up with their agencies, or meet with one of their classroom professors. Various arrangements were tried, and by the time the second cohort of students began their field practicum year, it was possible for all students to meet for group supervision at the school on a regular weekly basis, with individual contact occurring once or twice a semester, or more frequently if necessary.

Group Field Instruction Content

It was important to explain the purpose of the supervisory group to students, and particularly how this model of group field instruction was going to be different from the traditional model. It was emphasized that not only would each student be bringing his/her own knowledge, skills, and abilities in terms of life and work experience, but that they would be expected to share these experiences to help one another (Getzel, Goldberg, and Salmon, 1971; Steinberg, 2004). It was emphasized that this was an experiment, and that their input and cooperation would be an important factor in making this particular model of aging practice field instruction most helpful to them as part of their overall learning experience. The model could be changed if needed as we went along. However, it was made clear to all that students and the Field Instructor had a joint responsibility to try to make it work. Each participant was important, and valued.

> Being **valued** implies that group members have responsibility for each other and deal with each other at a certain level of authenticity. Unquestioning approval is not valuing. To some extent, in fact, it is the opposite. Valuing is based on a perception that the group needs its members–all of its members–in order to do its best work. (Ephross and Vassil, 1988)

GROUP PROCESS

Beginning Stage

Since the beginning stage of group development is particularly important, as it provides the foundation for what will follow (Kurland and Salmon, 1998), it was evident that there would be many challenges ahead. Students had little time outside of their full academic schedules, schedules as full-time employees, and full-time personal lives. In addition, beginnings were further disrupted by the impact of 9/11, which occurred right at the beginning of the first class's field practicum year.

However, even with all the problematic beginnings, students were able to start their field practicum year with a commitment to learn how to work more effectively with older individuals, and a connection to. one another with a camaraderie that enhanced the beginning of their field practicum group seminars.

The first class particularly felt special since they were aware that they were the initial class to participate in this pilot Aging and Health OYR Program. In addition, they had experienced a year of course work together, along with ongoing direction and intensive support provided by the PDC, prior to beginning their field practicum year. They thus entered this field work year with a beginning level of trust of one another and of the educational environment.

All students were required to write weekly process recordings and/or administrative logs and to reflect on their work on a regular basis. Not only were these recordings discussed in the field practicum seminar on a rotating basis, but the Field Instructor reviewed and responded in writing to them each week, raising questions, highlighting positive practice and/or administrative skills, and encouraging students to go forward and to risk.

During the beginning stage of the group, the role of the Field Instructor was to facilitate the group process to help build an environment of mutuality and trust, and to provide guidance and direction. Process recordings and administrative logs were used as the basis for seminar discussions. For example, administration and community organization students would present a summary of one of their fieldwork assignments. Some of the concerns presented were issues regarding start-up, student initiative as compared to agency oversight, supervisory difficulties, or clarification of a project. The student presenting would then ask the other seminar participants for feedback and particular support or information.

One of the first administrative issues presented in the group seminar was supervision of an employee whose attendance and behavior had become erratic and were affecting the services provided by the agency.

> ***Martha*** *said that supervision of this employee was one of her administrative assignments during her residency year of fieldwork. She said, "I don't know what to do with him; I can't count on him to show up and work on a regular basis." The **Field Instructor** said, "Let's look at that–but first we need to think about the seniors. That is always the first issue. Is his infrequent attendance hurting the seniors; is his behavior threatening to them?" **Martha** responded, "I don't*

*think they are affected by his absence yet but they will be. They have mentioned that sometimes he seems odd, different." One of her colleagues, **Joyce**, asked, "Is there any pattern to his behavior; for example, does he not show up at certain times of the month?" As **Martha** thought about it, she smiled and said, "yes, it is usually the beginning of the month; we have a regular special event and I particularly need him then." "Does he have a history of alcohol or drug abuse?" As **Martha** listened to her colleague's questions, she responded, "Yes, I think there is a history, but I thought he had stopped drinking." **Joyce** said, "Well, I think you might have a substance abuse problem here. Since this is my specialty, I can give you some help if you need it." Other seminar participants described experiences they had with drug abusing workers and other important issues of that kind. "What are you going to do, from an administrative point of view?" asked **Elaine**. **Jean** added, "That's right. I had to fire someone a while back, and my agency's policies were very helpful to me. Let's look at your agency policy, and figure out a way to confront the situation, using the policy as a way to get into the situation. That helps, because it is painful to open this up–for him, and hard for you, too–"*

Martha carefully listened to her colleagues and said that now she felt ready to go back to her agency and to begin to address this issue. She was able to use her colleagues' knowledge and experience to help her go forward in trying to find ways to help this troubled employee while at the same time knowing she had to explore and follow agency protocol.

Direct practice students presented an overview of a group or individual with whom they were working. They initially had difficulty asking for help from other group participants. They were experienced practitioners who were now being asked to discuss their direct practice work with their colleagues and to define their problem areas. In order to foster this process of mutual learning, it was important at the beginning of the group seminar process for the Field Instructor to help clarify and/or conceptualize issues for them. (For example, contracting was a major issue for students at the beginning of their field practicum year.)

One student, Deidre, had been assigned by her agency to work with an older male client, Mr. S, whom she would visit on a weekly basis in his home during her field practicum year. As she presented this client to her direct practice colleagues, it was apparent that neither she nor the agency was clear as to her role except to visit an isolated and lonely older gentleman.

*As **Deidre** said to her colleagues during the field practicum seminar, "I visit **Mr. S** and I don't know what to talk about." The **Field Instructor** reminded **Deidre** about the need to have a clear contract with clients. "Are you and **Mr. S** clear about your purpose in visiting him? What do you and/or the agency expect of your visit?" "Well, **Mr. S** has a meal delivered to him every day, and I guess one of the things I can talk to him about is his satisfaction with the meal." Since it seemed clear to the **Field Instructor** that **Deidre** was not clear how to move ahead in this relationship with **Mr. S**, she turned to the group: "Perhaps some of you can help Deidre as she struggles with her role with **Mr. S**. How might **Deidre** set a contract with **Mr. S**?" **Mary** asked **Deidre**, "What do you think **Mr. S** might want from your visit?" **Deidre** responded, "He is lonely and doesn't get out very much." Another student, **Edna**, said, "I found it real helpful to ask the client directly what he might want to talk about."*

*Another student, **Jean**, said, "I found it helpful to ask a client that was a man much like yours, directly. I tell you–it was like taking down a dam. (Laughing) He told me more than I wanted to hear–but it really was good."*

***Sara** asked, "Does he know how often you are coming, does he have any ideas as to how you might be helpful? Try asking him that." The **Field Instructor** then asked **Deidre** if she thought these suggestions might be useful. "I am not sure how it will work, but I think I can at least begin to talk with **Mr. S** I'll be direct and together we can begin to develop a contract for our work."*

The group had been helpful in encouraging Deidre to clarify her role with the client and to ask him how she might be helpful. Only then would they be able to establish a contract for the work to be completed. Developing a mutual contract occurred over many weeks. The worker continued to update her seminar colleagues about the process while they continued to provide feedback, support, and ideas to help her in this contracting process.

Learning to listen and to focus on clients' needs was a new and difficult challenge for students at the beginning of their field practicum year. With feedback and support from the group, they were able to move forward in developing their clinical skills. They began to assess overall needs of older individuals, which were often complex, and to develop a mutual contract as a way to focus on possible interventions. At the same time, students were encouraged to build on their years of social service experience by recognizing their own skills and knowledge, always trying to integrate field practice with the coursework. The Field Instructor's comments in the seminars, and the helpful participation of peers, were crucial. (See Shulman, 1999, for a discussion of the group as a mutual aid system.)

Middle Stage

By the end of the first semester and the completion of the first evaluation, students were ready to move into high gear. The group process was always moving forward. Thus, students were constantly challenged to keep up with one another. As they had become oriented to the group, and were clear about its purpose, they had begun to recognize commonalities among themselves, and had established norms of behavior. The group entered its middle stage (Kurland and Salmon, 1998).

In this phase, the students were able to relax more, and to begin to engage in the learning process through the use of mutual aid. They took a more active role in the group process and began to risk more with their colleagues. For example, the administration students raised ethical or troublesome situations they observed in their agencies and sought input from the group seminars. Case work and group work students used their process recordings as a means to seek feedback on their intervention skills and other ways to intervene and/or to assist particular clients. Students learned from one another about other service sites, different types of practice, different roles, organizational structures, types of clients, service needs, and cultural differences. The experiences of those in agencies with a mental health orientation were especially valuable for those students in case management agencies. They felt they were able to broaden their clinical understanding of their elderly clients, who had multiple needs, and thus be more effective in their work. Other students indicated that they had a better understanding of different policies and services of the varied settings by listening to their colleagues in the field supervision seminar. The mutual aid approach (Steinberg, 2004) was intrinsic to the learning that was achieved.

Administration students discussed a range of administrative issues, e.g., problematic workers, clients with dementia, how to write responses to an RFP (Request for Proposals), and how to facilitate executive meetings. However, the underlying focus always was on how they, as administrators, operated within the spectrum of agency services for the elderly, a complex and sometimes bewildering system. Students increasingly valued the support and information provided by their peers.

It was clear that the group had become, to some extent at least, a system of mutual support and mutual aid (Gitterman, 1989).

Casework and group work majors learned how to deal with client emotions, and how to intervene with a frail and/or homebound population. They discussed issues related to the terminally ill, how to apply the bio-psychosocial perspective and to adequately assess needs of clients, the importance of the process in practice (not just the outcome), and mental health concepts and clinical perspectives.

For the weekly meetings during this middle stage, students chose topics for discussion based on their process recordings; they also assumed more responsibility for interaction in the group. Time was spent discussing and clarifying differences between clinical social work and case management practice.

As it became clear that some students did not easily apply their beginning knowledge of clinical work to their actual involvement with clients, the Field Instructor decided to use role playing:

> *One of the students, **Linda**, talked during her presentation about how hard it was to talk about poor hygiene problems with one of her senior center members. "She really smells bad; other members are complaining and want me to do something about it. I don't know how to begin."*
>
> *The **Field Instructor** said, "**Linda**, let's try some role playing. This is really a very difficult situation and often a very common complaint in senior centers." When **Linda** agreed, the **Field Instructor** then said to the other seminar participants, "We need you to participate in role playing using some of your knowledge, skills, and experience to help **Linda** with this difficult practice situation."*
>
> *One of the students, **Melody**, who was more comfortable with her clinical skills, volunteered to assume the role of the social work interviewer. The **Field Instructor** said, "**Linda**, please play the role of **Ms. K**, since you know **Ms. K**, and none of us do." **Linda** was a little uncomfortable, but said, "Sure, I will try." **Melody** began by saying, "**Ms. K**, thank you for meeting with me today. Do you know why I asked to meet with you?" **Ms. K** said, "No, but it is nice to see you." "**Ms. K**, some of the people who share a table with you have complained about your hygiene." "My hygiene, what does that mean?" The **Field Instructor**, turning to another student, **Anne**, said, "**Anne**, why don't you pick up the role of the social worker at this point?" **Anne**, said, "**Ms. K**, have you noticed that some of the people at your table have moved away*

and won't sit next to you?" "Yes, but I don't understand why."
Anne *then took a deep breath and said, "They told me that you have a bad odor." **Ms. K** was very quiet for a moment, and then said, "But I don't understand why." At this point, the **Field Instructor** asked **Linda**, "How does it feel being the client, **Ms. K**?" "I feel bad–and I still don't know how to help her." The **Field Instructor** then suggested, "**Linda**, why don't we change roles and you become the worker. Perhaps you can practice some ways to be more comfortable in talking with **Ms. K**" "**Joan**, would you please take over the role of **Ms. K**?" **Joan** agreed. **Linda**, assuming her role as the worker, then picked up the conversation, "**Ms. K**, I am sorry I made you feel bad. But I want to help you. Do you know any reason why people might say you smell bad?" **Joan**, in her role of **Ms. K**, answered, "No, but maybe if I talk to my doctor, he might know why. I shower every day, really." **Linda** then ventured, "Perhaps I can go to the doctor with you. Would that be okay?" **Joan**, in the role of **Ms. K**, smiled and said, "Yes, that would be good. Thank you."*

Many different approaches were tried. Students who played the client also began to realize which questions or comments were helpful and which were hurtful. The Field Instructor not only kept the role playing on track, and encouraged all the students to participate in one role or the other, but also helped students identify what seemed to work for them–either from the client's perspective or from that of the worker. Playing the role of her client with poor hygiene seemed to help particularly the senior center worker. She saw her colleagues struggle with their role as helper in this difficlt situation, but she also experienced some of their clinical skills as they demonstrated how to work with and form a helping relationship with the client.

The use of the group model for field instruction also provided a valuable opportunity for all students to experience being in a mutual aid group. Most students were not group work majors, but many of them did work in group settings, such as senior centers or adult day care programs. Through their involvement in the field practicum group seminar, they were exposed to group process and began to have a more intimate understanding of how a group experience can be useful for older adults, particularly those individuals who are alone and seeking opportunities for socialization with others. Such knowledge would be helpful to them as they developed and implemented groups in their social service agencies. Participation in the field instruction group seminar enabled all students to have the opportunity to observe and reflect on their group experience.

Ending Stage

As the field practicum year approached its ending stage, it was clear that the students had begun to feel a sense of comfort and ease with one another (Kurland and Salmon, 1998). They had entered wholeheartedly into the group process, had risked personal information about themselves and their agencies, had become aware of different skills and types of programs serving older individuals and their families, and looked forward to this special time together.

At the end of the second semester, the completion of their field practicum year, students were all asked to write a summary of their student/work experiences, both as a way to help them see what they had learned and to enhance awareness of their own growth and development. They summarized each of their aging-oriented assignments, the number of sessions, contacts, meetings, etc., and what had been accomplished. Furthermore, they used this summary to discuss their role in the work and what they had learned about providing services to older individuals. They discussed what their approach to practice was, now, after the year of the field practicum. This summary was included as part of their involvement in the final evaluation process.

EVALUATION

The "Aging and Health" Program was new in many ways, and several evaluation mechanisms were devised to provide indications of those aspects that were successful and those that needed change. Among the types of evaluation used, two–focus groups and a telephone survey–bore directly on the group model of field instruction.

Focus Groups

Since this was an experimental model of group field instruction, it was important for everyone involved to get a sense of what worked well and what did not. As part of the ending stage of the group process, focus groups were conducted. There was a focus group for Task

Supervisors and Administrators of the participating agencies, and there were two separate focus groups for students.

Task Supervisor/Administrator Focus Group

The focus group held at the end of the field practicum year for Task Supervisors and Administrators produced comments indicating that the Aging and Health Program was an "incredible and wonderful" opportunity for students above and beyond the traditional OYR program. Task Supervisors also talked about the complex projects and assignments related to aging services that students had undertaken and completed successfully as part of their fieldwork. One common theme was that the students had learned to be more independent and to think on their own. Students had enriched their agencies while in the program, as they often brought back learning about aging individuals and their needs for services from the classroom and field instruction seminar to the agency. They became the informed gerontologists for the future.

The Task Supervisors and Administrators felt that the group field instruction model had saved time and freed up agency supervisors for other tasks. Also, conflict between agency personnel and the student decreased, since the HCCSW Field Instructor was the one guiding the student's learning tasks.

Student Focus Groups

In the focus group for administration students, they immediately talked about their fieldwork placements and the challenges that their assignments represented. One student commented: "Being a seasoned professional, it was hard to be a learner. I was working on a project with a local committee . . . I had never done anything like that before . . . There were many responsibilities . . . the field supervision group was really useful . . . My colleagues helped me solve problems. They supported me in providing leadership to the committee which was able to develop a resource guide for caregivers of elders."

Another student said, "We now try to see behind the presenting problem. Because of how I do social work with older people now, others in my agency can see the potential of social work practice."

The casework and group work students valued the case presentations that were made during the field instruction seminar and the suggestions from their colleagues: "We gave each other feedback and that helped us and the clients." They also valued the use of process recordings. Others said they learned how to summarize their work with older adults and their families, that it gave them a chance to step back, to focus more on clinical issues, to analyze their work, to find clients' strengths and their own strengths, and to further examine their own learning needs.

With respect to the group field instruction process itself, students said, "We brought our issues in from the field of aging services and we received support from the instructor and the other students." "We learned to be better workers for our older clients." "We learned about mutual aid." Also, "The group should be a tool to help students deal with stress, give support, learn things and reflect on your growth."

Telephone Interviews

In order to determine the students' perceptions of the effect the Aging and Health Program had on their knowledge and skills, as well as on their clients' lives, a telephone interview survey was conducted in December 2003. All 29 students were interviewed. The results indicated that the students worked in a variety of agencies serving community-dwelling older adults, their families, and their caregivers. These included senior centers, Alzheimer's programs, home care, elder abuse/crime prevention programs, hospitals, senior housing adult day health and substance abuse treatment. The clients served were of diverse backgrounds (29% African-American or Caribbean-American, 27% Latino, 5% Asian, 33% Caucasian, and 3% recent Russian immigrants); a total of 64% of clients served were minority and/or immigrant elders. Two-thirds of clients served had "poor" health; 15% had "fair" health status; only 19% were in "good" health. Half of the clients served were poor, one-fourth were of "lower-middle" income, and the remainder were middle-class.

When asked which component of their social work education had helped the most in their work with older people, 72% of graduates and current students listed "Field Instructor." This ranked second only to "special courses" (76%). When asked what they had gotten from the Aging and Health Program that has made it possible to improve the quality of their clients' lives, "Field Instruction/Field Instructor" was at the top of the list (45% of respondents). Students and graduates mentioned many times that the "support, peer group and networking" provided by the program (particularly in the group Field Instruction Seminar) and by the Professional Development Counselor were "special" and that the "peer learning, sharing" and "nurturance/guidance" were key in their ability to provide better services to older clients, use improved administrative/supervisory skills, and deal better with differential needs of elderly clients, families and caregivers.

CONCLUSION

One of the primary benefits of group work is the development of mutual aid (Northen and Kurland, 2001). This model of group field instruction was no exception. Students began to recognize individual skill levels, levels of competence, experience, and responsibilities, and they were able to use the mutual aid process to grow and to learn in their work with older adults and their families.

The students had learned about different types of aging practice and settings, and had begun to learn from one another about different types of practice skills, how to analyze their work, and to respond to difficult situations. They learned how to use one another for support, information, growth, and honesty.

Experienced in social service work and with a commitment to working with older people and their families, students entered their graduate social work education ready to move forward and develop professional skills. The field practicum, and group field instruction, became the place where each student could bring experience, knowledge and a quest for new learning–and learn from and be challenged by other students–in a safe environment.

As these students moved toward the completion of their graduate social work studies, they became part of a network of professional aging service providers who can reach out to each other throughout their careers for support, ideas, information, resources, and camaraderie. As tomorrow's leaders in gerontological social work, the hope is that they will be able to use these formative connections to influence social policy and to assure quality of care for those older individuals most in need of professional social work services.

The development of a group model of field instruction in the "Aging and Health" Program, an innovative work-study MSW program, occurred in part due to necessity and, in part, because of the belief by all Program personnel in the efficacy of the group model in learning and in fostering communication, support, and cohesiveness among the students. Despite difficulties in the beginning stage, both groups proceeded through their year-long process of enhancing student learning and integration of classroom and practice, with favorable results. The educational experiences of this program have provided Aging and

Health work-study students an opportunity to provide better services to community-based older individuals needing social work intervention. Evaluation by both students and agency personnel has indicated strong support for the group model of field instruction and the school-based Field Instructor.

This group work model of field instruction is one attempt to address the diverse and changing needs of students, agencies, and social work schools. Students are exposed to different types of social service settings and the wide range of needs of elderly clients and their families. The group setting provides an opportunity for mutual support as well as a time to test individual knowledge and skills within an educational environment that is separate from students' social service agencies and work-a-day worlds. There are many challenges to be addressed by such a model: logistics of time, different agency settings and task supervisors, and different student learning styles, among others. However, based on the experiences of the past two cohorts of Aging and Health students, it is evident that the group process has the power to foster learning, and to forge strong bonds among very diverse individuals as they become the next generation of gerontological social work practitioners.

REFERENCES

Abels, Paul A. (1983). On the Nature of Supervision: The Medium is the Group. In H. Weissman, I. Epstein, and A. Savage. *Agency Based Social Work: Neglected Aspects of Clinical Practice* (pp. 250-258). Philadelphia: Temple University Press.

Ephross, Paul H., and Vassil, Thomas, V. (1988). *Groups That Work: Structure and Process.* New York: Columbia University Press, p. 47.

Getzel, G., Goldberg, J., and Salmon, R. (1971). Supervising in Groups as a Model for Today. *Social Casework, 52*(3), 154-163.

Getzel, G., and Salmon, R. (1985). Group Supervision: An Organizational Approach. *The Clinical Supervisor, 3*(1), 27-43.

Gitterman, A. (1989). Building Mutual Support in Groups. *Social Work with Groups, 12*(2), 5-21.

Graziano, R., Salmon, R., and Berman, E. (2002). Using a Group Work Approach to Develop the Potential of Students in a Non-Traditional MSW/Work Study Program. *Journal of Teaching in Social Work, 22*(3/4), 71-88.

Haffey, M., and Starr, R. (1988). *Designing a Work Study Program: When Social Service Employment Meets Professional Educator.* New York: The Lois & Samuel Silberman Fund.

Kaplan, T. (1988). Group Field Instruction: Rationale and Practical Application. *Social Work with Groups, 11*(1/2), 125-143.

Kurland, R., and Salmon, R. (1998). *Teaching a Methods Course in Social Work with Groups.* Alexandria, VA: Council on Social Work Education.

Marshack, E., and Glassman, U. (1991). Innovative Models for Field Instruction: Departing from Traditional Methods. In D. Schneck, B. Grossman, and U. Glassman (Eds.), *Field Education in Social Work: Contemporary Issues and Trends* (pp. 84-95). Dubuque, IA: Kendall/Hunt Publishing Company.

Northen, H., and Kurland, R. (2001). *Social Work with Groups* (3rd ed.). New York: Columbia University Press.

Potts, M. K. (1992). Adjustment of Graduate Students to the Educational Process: Effects of Part-Time Enrollment and Extra-Curricular Roles. *Journal of Continuing Social Work Education,* 28(1), 61-76.

Salmon, R., and Walker, J. (1981). The One Year Residence Program: An Alternative Path to the Master's Degree in Social Work. *Journal of Education for Social Work,* 17(1), 21-29.

Salmon, R., Haffey, M., Blau, S., and Johnson, D. (1993). The Potential for Staff Development Through Work-Study Programs. *Journal of Continuing Social Work Education,* 5(4), 23-28.

Shulman, L. (1999). *The Skills of Helping Individuals, Families, Groups, and Communities, 4th ed.* Itasca, IL: F.E. Peacock Publishers, Inc., pp. 302-318.

Shulman, L. (1993). *Interactional Supervision.* Washington, DC: NASW Press.

Steinberg, D. (2004). *The Mutual Aid Approach to Working with Groups: Helping People Help Each Other* (2nd ed.). Binghamton, NY: The Haworth Press, Inc.

The Use of a Mutual Aid Group
with Home Attendants

Sister Maria Theresa Amato, OP, MSW

SUMMARY. This article reflects the experience of six home attendants whose clients were individuals diagnosed with Alzheimer's and other related dementias. It examines how they used a mutual aid group to discuss the stresses, professional and personal problems that resulted from their work. *[Article copies available for a fee from The Haworth Document Delivery Service: 1-800-HAWORTH. E-mail address: <docdelivery@haworthpress.com> Website: <http://www.HaworthPress.com> © 2004 by The Haworth Press, Inc. All rights reserved.]*

KEYWORDS. Adult day-care, Alzheimer's and related dementia diseases, empowerment, mutual aid group, care-giving, care-giver stress/fatigue

Home attendants are a terribly neglected profession. They do difficult and often complex work and receive little appreciation or monetary compensation. They have little opportunity to express their needs or to be recognized for their professionalism. In New York City, most of the professional home-care workers are Black and Hispanic women. De-

[Haworth co-indexing entry note]: "The Use of a Mutual Aid Group with Home Attendants." Amato, Sister Maria Theresa. Co-published simultaneously in *Journal of Gerontological Social Work* (The Haworth Social Work Practice Press, an imprint of The Haworth Press, Inc.) Vol. 44, No. 1/2, 2004, pp. 243-253; and: *Group Work and Aging: Issues in Practice, Research, and Education* (ed: Robert Salmon, and Roberta Graziano) The Haworth Social Work Practice Press, an imprint of The Haworth Press, Inc., 2004, pp. 243-253. Single or multiple copies of this article are available for a fee from The Haworth Document Delivery Service [1-800-HAWORTH, 9:00 a.m. - 5:00 p.m. (EST). E-mail address: docdelivery@haworthpress.com].

spite attention to racism and sexism, women still make up 90% of the home attendant workers in this country (Donovan, 1987).

This article is based on the author's work with a group for home attendants who came to an adult day-care program with their clients who had been diagnosed with Alzheimer's or other related dementia and who formed a mutual aid group. The purpose of this group was to improve the home attendants' working relationship with their clients and their families. It was the author's belief that having a time and place to discuss the stresses, issues and problems that they would encounter working as home attendants might lead to positive change.

REVIEW OF THE LITERATURE

The demographic trend within the United States with respect to aging indicates that the number of elderly persons has increased by 60% since the 1970s (Donovan, Kurzman, & Rotman, 1993; Burbridge, 1993). According to the U.S. Bureau of the Census (2000), life expectancy will increase from 77.6 in the year 2000 to 82.6 in 2050. By the year 2010, the "Baby Boomer" generation will reach age 65 and over. The projections indicate that by 2030, the population aged 65 and older will grow to approximately 70 million, an increase of 100% over 30 years. Individuals over the age of 85 are more likely to suffer illness and disability and will be in need of long-term care (Donovan, Kurzman, & Rotman, 1993).

The demand for home attendants and home health aides has consistently increased over the last decade (Donovan, 1987; Ebenstein, 1998). A number of factors are responsible for this increase. Home care has become a substitute for nursing home or hospice care. Many elderly and disabled persons prefer to remain at home even as their physical and cognitive functioning decline. Through services provided by the government at the federal, state, and local levels, such as home health care services, older and/or disabled individuals can live at home while maintaining a sense of independence and self-sufficiency, both of which are often hindered in institutional settings.

There has been a shift away from the elderly depending on their children, particularly women within the family or other female relatives, to paid home-care workers. Many of these previously available female family members are now part of the work force. Additionally, there has been a decrease in family size; fewer children are in a position to act as caregivers to aging parents (Burbridge, 1993; Donovan, Kurzman, & Rotman, 1993).

The rapidly expanding home-care industry is emerging as a major source of employment for low-income minority women in the United States (Donovan, 1987). A large percentage of home attendants are Black American women and/or recent immigrant women from the Caribbean and Latin American countries. These women are often their family's primary wage earners. A significant number of them do not have high school diplomas. Many of the problems that home-care workers face are deeply rooted in racism, sexism and the economic inequalities of society. These workers may be treated disparagingly, micromanaged by their clients or their client's family members, or pressed to perform tasks not in their job description such as washing windows, shampooing rugs, or caring for a client's pets (Chichin & Cantor, 1992).

Literature indicates a broad range of frustration and problems that home-care workers must confront within their daily jobs. These include conflicting instructions from family members, working alone without peer support and receiving low wages with limited or no medical coverage or other fringe benefits (Feldman, 1993; Bartoldus, Gillery, & Sturges, 1989). Home attendants also receive training and supervision that are inadequate, are often discriminated against on the basis of race, gender and/or nationality, and are verbally and/or physically abused by clients as a result of the Alzheimer's or related dementia disease from which they suffer. Workers routinely deal with emotionally demanding and highly charged situations that can result in significantly elevated levels of stress. Many spend their time with dependent and needy clients only to return home to perform care-giving tasks necessary to maintain their own family's needs (Chicin, 1991; Donovan, 1987; Donovan, Kurzman, & Rotman, 1993; Eustis, Kane, & Fischer, 1993).

The home attendants' support group described in this article utilized a mutual aid approach. Mutual aid refers to people helping one another as they think things through (Steinberg, 2003). In this group, members helped one another by utilizing their own experiences and acquired knowledge. Each member of the group had something to contribute. Working collaboratively, these women shared ideas, experiences and feelings as they worked collectively, utilizing a problem-solving process (Northen & Kurland, 2001).

The clients the group members served were from White, Italian and Jewish middle-class backgrounds. Six home attendants participated in the group: two women were from Jamaica (Wilma & Edna), one was from Trinidad (Julie), another was from Italy (Rosa), one from Haiti

(Joan), and the last was from Norway (Maryann). These women had been accompanying their clients to the Alzheimer's Adult Day Care Program from six months to three years.

The purpose of the group was to help the home attendants work more effectively with their clients and their clients' families. The group provided an opportunity for these professionals to discuss their varied concerns and frustrations as they cared for their clients, in addition to any problems that might evolve regarding the clients' family members.

These women frequently dealt with the racially prejudicial attitudes held by their clients' families or by the clients themselves. These prejudices might not be blatantly expressed, but were subtly revealed. For example, a client or a family member might follow the home attendant around the house to make sure nothing was stolen. Burghardt (1982) indicates that all individuals possess subtle forms of personal oppression and bias and that racism, sexism, and classism are found in many forms in our society. The members of the home attendants' group did experience these, as will be discussed in this paper. In fact, the oppression and racism that the home attendants experienced were instrumental in leading to the formation of the home attendants' support group.

The members of the home attendants' support group worked with clients in the latter stages of Alzheimer's/dementia disease who exhibited various cognitive difficulties. These clients repeated queries, and exhibited an inability to organize events, days of the week, seasons of the year and people, whether family members or others. Their functional capacity became compromised as they tried to perform activities of daily life. The clients relied on their home attendants to tend to their personal needs: preparing meals, doing laundry, shopping, cleaning, bathing and dressing them, providing oral care, feeding them, and, when they became incontinent, changing their diapers. The clients often manifested behavioral problems such as anger and hostility. Sometimes they were threatening and they could be verbally or physically abusive to the home attendant. They tended to pace or run away from their caregivers, looking for what they considered "home" or a familiar space. As the disease progressed, the clients had increased difficulty being understood. There was an overt breakdown in ability to articulate speech and stuttering often occurred, and the client increasingly created new words or expressions. Given the client's behaviors, the job was not easy for the attendants. They needed to express concern, compassion, and tolerance, even in the face of the clients' negative behaviors (Reisberg & Franssen, 1999).

The group described here helped the home attendants in four major ways. First, it provided support, allowing for sharing of feelings, frustrations, and concerns. Second, it enabled its members to learn from each other's experiences, techniques, and skills. Third, the group empowered its members. Fourth, it provided its members with an ongoing sense of community.

SUPPORT AND THE SHARING OF FEELINGS AND CONCERNS

Before the group began, the home attendants indicated that they had no one they could speak with regarding issues and frustrations that came up at work. They expressed their desire to share these experiences with people who were in similar situations and who therefore would understand their problems. The home attendants expressed a need to be heard, to interact with others in order to be challenged, validated, and affirmed.

> Rosa's client's spouse, Mario, has been described as impatient, determined, and demanding. He believes that "the man is the head of the household and what he says goes." When Rosa went to bathe her client, she found black and blue marks on the client's back. When she brought this to the attention of Mario, she was informed that the client lost her balance and bumped into something. In the group, Rosa expressed her fear that the client was being physically abused. Rosa was already concerned about Mario's yelling and cursing and that his wife was already a victim of verbal and now possibly physical abuse.

In expressing her concerns to the group, Rosa was able to express her fear for the client's safety as well as her own. The group helped her to express her apprehension about being falsely accused of physically hurting her client. Rosa stated that she felt isolated. She could not tell her own family due to the issue of confidentiality; additionally, her spouse and children would want her to leave this job that she loved doing. The group gave Rosa the time and a safe space to discuss this issue. She felt affirmed by the group and as the other members listened, Rosa expressed her feelings without sensing any judgmental or disapproving tone. As the discussion continued, suggestions were made by the group members at Rosa's request, since she sought insight into the problems that she presented. Rosa needed to take the information home and process what was shared.

The following week Rosa addressed the group and thanked them for their help. She informed the group about the methods she had begun to use to monitor and hopefully change the abusive behavior.

> Rosa stated that she now keeps a written record of any bruises or scratches on the client's body. She let Mario know that she had found the marks. Rosa gave a great deal of thought to the discussion that had taken place in the group regarding Mario's denial about his wife having Alzheimer's disease as well as his lack of understanding about the disease. Rosa recalled that Mario enjoyed reading and often quoted articles to her. With a gleam in her eyes she explained to the group how she brought the book *The 36 Hour Day* (by Mace & Rabins, 1999) to Mario and how she explained to him that she used the book to help her understand the client's behavior. Mario looked through the book and asked that she loan it to him to read. One of the group members, Wilma, with a bit of sarcasm in her voice, said "It probably will just sit there on the table where you left it and collect dust." Rosa, laughing, said, "Wilma, to tell you the truth, I thought that too, but to my surprise I found the book moved to the table next to where Mario sits in the living room."

The group discussion motivated and empowered Rosa to take action to alleviate her fears and concerns regarding her client. She took steps to monitor and prevent any further abuse. Mario began to ask Rosa questions about how she manages to get his wife to respond to her. Rosa indicated that Mario is now attempting to understand the nature of the disease and begin to deal with his denial. The group affirmed Rosa's handling of this important situation. Rosa was able to penetrate the core of Mario's roughness and impatience with his wife. Mario had been feeling that he was losing control as his wife's disease worsened.

LEARNING FROM OTHERS' EXPERIENCES

At another group meeting, Maryann allowed members to provide support to her. As a result, she was able to learn from the experiences of the other workers. At times she, too, needed to be challenged to look at her past experiences with her client and take the time to process her thoughts and feelings to determine if she wanted to be a home attendant for a woman, Flora, who had been a personal friend for years before she began showing signs of Alzheimer's disease.

Maryann worked as a Nanny for 15 years for Flora's daughter's three children. During that time, she had become friends with Flora since she frequently visited Flora's daughter and grandchildren. Maryann was the newest member of the group. Her client, Flora, was diagnosed with middle stage Alzheimer's. At the second meeting of the group, Maryann took a big risk. She had admitted to the group that Flora was refusing to bathe herself. "I know what to do with children, but how do I get a grown woman to wash herself?" Maryann asked.

Her question was the beginning of Maryann's becoming a "real" member of the group. The other members expressed their own experiences and openly discussed the techniques that they had learned. One in particular, shared by Edna, helped Maryann to relax and join the others in laughter.

In a heavy Jamaican accent Edna noted, "I once had a client who would not take a bath no matter what I did. My client was at the point where she refused to sponge bathe or even change her clothes." The group members focused on Edna, waiting to hear her solution to the problem. Edna said "Well, girl, I asked her daughter what her mother liked to do that involved water and she said that her mother loved to go to the beach. Well, that night on my way home, I bought a cooler, shovel pail, and watering can. The next morning I wore my bathing suit under my uniform. I put a beach chair in the shower and dressed the client in her suit and gave her the cooler, pail and watering can. We entered the shower together and pretended we were on the beach. It took time but eventually my client let me bathe her." Amidst the laughter of the group, Maryann could be heard saying, "I guess I have to invest in a nice bathing suit."

Maryann thanked the group for listening and for helping her. She appreciated the group members' reaching out to her and affirming her concerns about her lack of training, without putting her down. This interaction paved the way to Maryann's acceptance by the other group members, all of whom had a great deal more experience than Maryann did.

EMPOWERMENT OF GROUP MEMBERS

Several weeks later, Maryann came back to the group with a serious issue. Once again she called upon the group for support and advice.

"I'm having difficulty with my client's daughter Terry, whom I find unsupportive and in denial of her mother's illness,' she said. 'Terry takes advantage of me, she is placing more and more responsibility for caring for her mother on me as she pulls away and gets more involved in her own career and in that of her husband."

The group listened intently and acknowledged Maryann's feelings of anger and frustration. Joan replied, "Terry seems to have no regard for what you might be doing or what your needs are." The rest of the members nodded affirmatively.

Maryann continued to explain that during the course of a phone conversation with Terry, she became aware that Terry had not visited her mother or spoken with her over the weekend, when Maryann was off. In an angry voice, Maryann said, "Terry lives a half a mile away from her mother. Neither she nor her children checked on her mother, or brought her a meal for the whole weekend. She still thinks that her mother can care for herself." Maryann described that when she got to Flora's home on Monday, she found her in the same clothes she had been wearing the previous Friday. Flora had not bathed or brushed her teeth and had not taken her medication. From what she could observe the client must have eaten some bread and a few pieces of ham that had been left in the refrigerator on Friday. Terry was to have done the food shopping for her mother that night, but had not done so. Maryann had to calm Flora down, give her medication, clean, and feed her. Maryann decided that she would meet with Terry and inform her about the neglect that she witnessed.

Edna gave Maryann some advice: "It appears that Flora is getting worse, she needs to have coverage 24 hours per day. Her safety is at risk. Watch out that Terry does not try to increase your hours." Rosa chimed in, reminding Maryann about her previous conversation regarding her own health problems: her high blood pressure and bad back, and how her own children were very concerned that she was putting her own health in jeopardy. Maryann decided that she would draw up a contract, stating exactly what her hours and responsibilities were so that she would not be overwhelmed or taken advantage of by Flora's family.

Maryann now remembered how in the beginning she had felt inadequate because of her lack of formal training and understanding of Alzheimer's disease. With the group's guidance, based on their own training and experience, Maryann had a place to bring up how to go about confronting the client's daughter. The group members acknowledged Maryann's needs and listened to her as she worked through the problem before her. The group members helped Maryann obtain the confidence she needed to feel empowered to speak on her client's behalf as the client was unable to speak or to advocate for herself.

SENSE OF COMMUNITY

The sense of community that the group provided for its members was illustrated in several ways. The women went beyond discussing the emotional and physical demands of their job. They shared the happy events and stressful concerns of their private lives.

Joan's father needed heart surgery. She wanted her father to be treated in an American hospital. Joan informed the group of the deplorable medical conditions in Haiti and that she would do anything to bring her father here. Joan spent all the money that she had in the bank to pay for her father's plane ticket to America and to help her mother and siblings with the expenses that would be incurred while her father was here. As the end of the month came closer, she found that she had insufficient funds, and she could not pay all of her rent. Wilma shared this information with the group and a collection was taken to help Joan meet this expense.

On another occasion, Wilma was not her usual self. She appeared to be preoccupied. Edna made mention of it to her and asked if she would like to share what was bothering her. Wilma expressed her concern over her daughter who is a diabetic and was informed during her recent examination that her kidney was not functioning properly. She now has to go for a special test. "I'm so afraid that she will have to put on dialysis," she said. The group members offered support and concern. They assured her of their prayers for her daughter and herself during this stressful time, for which Wilma expressed her appreciation, saying that she believes in the power of prayer.

The group also shared the happy events of life. Birthdays and holidays were a time to celebrate. Music and food from the various ethnic cultures were shared and recipes were exchanged. The stories of how each culture celebrated their holidays were told and a better understanding and sensitivity of each ethnic group were established among them.

CONCLUSIONS AND IMPLICATIONS

The home attendants' mutual aid group was clearly successful. The group provided these paraprofessionals with a common safe space and the time in which they could express their thoughts, concerns, questions, and fears. The women realized that the first issues to be addressed by the group were racial and ethnic prejudices. They first had to deal with the differences among themselves within the group itself and then reckon with the racial and ethnic innuendoes that surfaced and were manifested in their day-to-day interactions with the families and clients to whom they were assigned. These six women experienced the value of learning from each other, as they worked collectively through the problem-solving process. The result was that they were able to speak openly, give and receive advice from each other in a nonjudgmental, trusting atmosphere. These women acknowledged their differences, recognized their common experiences, and were able to lighten their burden, relieve their stress, and thus become better caregivers.

With the demand for home attendants to serve our increasing elderly population, group work using a mutual aid approach is a means through which home attendants can be encouraged, experience empathy, and gain interpersonal growth and understanding of their shared profession. The use of the mutual aid process can be a means of bringing about healing and freeing individuals to express their opinions. The collaborative problem-solving process can nurture group members, enhance decision-making and build more cohesiveness (Northen & Kurland, 2001). Mutual aid groups for home attendants could be utilized in Adult Day Care programs, vendor agencies, nursing homes, and even hospitals. This type of group could decrease burnout and enhance job performance.

REFERENCES

Bartoldus, E., Gillery, B., & Sturges, P. (1989). "Job Related Stress and Coping among Home Care Workers with Elderly People." *Health and Social Work*, 14 (3), 204-210.

Burbridge, L. (1993). "The Labor Market for Home Care Workers: Demand, Supply, and Institutional Barriers." *The Gerontologist*, 33 (1), 41-46.

Burghardt, S. (1982). *The Other Side of Organizing*. Schenkman Publishing Co., Cambridge, MA.

Chichin, E. (1991). The Treatment of Paraprofessional Workers in the Home. *Pride Journal of Long Term Home Health Care*, 10 (1), 26-35.

Chichin, E.R., & Cantor, M.H. (1992). "The Home Care Industry: Strategies for Survival in an Era of Dwindling Resources." *Journal of Aging & Social Policy*, 4 (1/2), 89-105.

Donovan, R. (1987). Home Care Work: A Legacy of Slavery in U.S. Health Care. *Affilia*, 2 (3).

Donovan, R., Kurzman, P., & Rotman, C. (1993). "Improving the Lives of Home Care Workers: A Partnership of Social Work and Labor." *Social Work*, 38 (5), 579-585.

Ebenstein, H. (1998). They Were Once Like Us: Learning from Home Care Workers Who Care for the Elderly. *Journal of Gerontological Social Work,* 30 (3/4) 191-201.

Eustis, N., Kane, R., & Fischer, L. (1993). Home Care Quality and the Home Care Worker Beyond Quality Assurance as Usual. *The Gerontologist*, 33 (1), 64-73.

Feldman, P. (1993). "Work Life Improvements for Home Care Workers, Impact and Feasibility." *The Gerontologist*, 33 (1), 47-54.

Mace, N., & Rabins, P. (1999). *The 36 Hour Day* (3rd ed.). The John Hopkins University Press, Baltimore & London.

Northen, H., & Kurland, R. (2001). *Social Work with Groups* (3rd ed.). Columbia University Press.

Reisberg, B., & Franssen, E. (1999). *The Encyclopedia of Visual Medicine Series an Atlas of Alzheimer's Disease*. Parthenon, Pearl River, NY.

Steinberg, D.M. (2003). "Mutual Aid and Social Justice," in Sullivan, N., Mesbur, E., Lang, N., Goodman, D., & Mitchell, L. *Social Work with Groups Social Justice through Personal Community Societal Change*. Binghamton, NY: The Haworth Press, Inc., 91-99.

U.S. Administration on Aging Web Page: *http://www.aoa.gov/aoa/stats/profile*. July 2000.

Remembering
With and Without Awareness
Through Poetry
to Better Understand Aging and Disability

Andrew Malekoff, MSW

SUMMARY. Poetry has been described as a universal translator. I offer three poems that are evocative of my experience as a child with my grandfathers and their disabilities; and as an adult attempting to deal with the impending death of my father. My wish is that the first poem will reinforce the idea that connecting with one's own memories of aged and disabled family members might support our interactions with people who are aged and disabled in the here and now. I present the final two poems to encourage those working with family members of seriously ill aged people in a hospital setting to better understand the stress of decision-making and to consider devising short-term mutual aid groups to support them during a time for which no preparation exists. *[Article copies available for a fee from The Haworth Document Delivery Service: 1-800-HAWORTH. E-mail address: <docdelivery@haworthpress.com> Website: <http://www.HaworthPress.com> © 2004 by The Haworth Press, Inc. All rights reserved.]*

[Haworth co-indexing entry note]: "Remembering With and Without Awareness Through Poetry to Better Understand Aging and Disability." Malekoff, Andrew. Co-published simultaneously in *Journal of Gerontological Social Work* (The Haworth Social Work Practice Press, an imprint of The Haworth Press, Inc.) Vol. 44. No. 1/2, 2004, pp. 255-264; and: *Group Work and Aging: Issues in Practice, Research, and Education* (ed: Robert Salmon, and Roberta Graziano) The Haworth Social Work Practice Press, an imprint of The Haworth Press, Inc., 2004, pp. 255-264. Single or multiple copies of this article are available for a fee from The Haworth Document Delivery Service [1-800-HAWORTH, 9:00 a.m. - 5:00 p.m. (EST). E-mail address: docdelivery@haworthpress.com].

KEYWORDS. Aging, disability, short-term groups, mutual aid, poetry

INTRODUCTION: REMEMBERING WITHOUT AWARENESS

Remembering without awareness is a phrase I really like. It is not as fancy as the psychoanalytic terms transference or countertransference and not as abstruse as, "It's déjà vu all over again," a line attributed to Yogi Berra. Nevertheless, all of these terms and phrases are in the same ballpark. They connote something that is evoked in us in the present with roots in the past that has escaped our present awareness.

REMEMBERING MY GRANDFATHERS' DISABILITIES

I don't remember a great deal about my grandfathers. What I do remember is that they loved me and that they had disabilities and prostheses. Grandpa Harry had both his legs amputated due to diabetes and Grandpa Joe had a glass eye, the result of a carpentry accident. As a child, their disabilities were never hidden from me. I went with my dad and Grandpa Harry when he had one of his prosthetic legs fitted, and Grandpa Joe regularly took his eye out and showed it to me at my request. And I remember seeing Grandpa Joe, who I called Pop, tied down to a hospital bed when he was dying, a scene that I relived many years later with my mother.

In my first year of graduate school, although I was interested in working with youth, I was placed in a crisis intervention program for the aged. I made home visits to people who were blind, bedridden, slow afoot, and terminally ill. And I worked with a group in a Senior Center where there was a member whose main goal was to get the Center to order a certain salt-free salad dressing. The other members thought he was a pest. I loved his spirit and thought he was a great advocate.

I was surprised at how well I connected with all of the older people I got to know that year when I was 26-years-old. Although I should not have been surprised. As I later realized, I was remembering without awareness my short time together with my grandpas. And what I learned from those relationships was tolerance and understanding for disability and aging. It was only years later, through poetry, that many of these memories were recalled *with awareness*. Our early memories and recollections, whether or not we are aware of them, influence how we relate in the present. Poetry helps me to remember not only the people and times but the texture of our time together.

Poetry I.

bow-wow

when i
was
2 years
old
i had a
bow-wow:

> not a
> real dog
> but
> a fake
> one.

one
day
when
riding
home
from
the
beach, i
threw
him out
the car
win-dough.

i
started
to
laugh.

then
i
cried.

my
grandpas
convinced

my
daddy
to
stop
the
car
and
turn
around
to
retrieve
my
bow-wow.

my
grandpas
were
cool
guys.

one
of
them
had
a
wooden
leg.

the
other
one
had
a
glass
eye.

nobody
would
tell

how
they
got
them.

i
wondered
what
fake
parts
i'd
have
when
i
got
old.

maybe
i'd
have
a
rubber
hand
that
i'd
screw
into
my
wrist.

maybe
i
wouldn't
screw
it
in
so
good
so
that

when
people
shook
hands
with
me
it'd
fall
off
my
arm.

i
wondered
if
they'd
be
as
surprised
as
i
was
the
first
time
grandpa
took
out
his
eye
and
put
it
in
a
cup.

i
remember
asking

grandpa
if
he
could
still
see
me
through
his
eye
once
he
took
it
out
of
his
head.

anyway,
after
i
threw
my
bow-wow
out
of
the
win-dough
for
the
third
time
my
dad
refused
to
turn
the
car

around
to
fetch
him,
        even
        though
        my
        grandpas
        tried
        to
        convince
        him
        one
        last
        time.

i
fell
asleep
and
dreamt
that
the
buzzards
swooped
down
and
ripped
my
bow-wow's
ears
off
his
head.

and
then
my
grandpas
came

back
to
get
him.

they
took
him
to
a
toy
store.

they
bought
mr. potato head
and
gave
my

bow-wow
his
ears.

like
i
said,
my
grandpas
were
cool
guys

as
far
as
i
can
remember.

REMEMBERING MY FATHER DYING

Of course I never knew, when I knew my grandfathers, that one day I would be dealing with my parents' aging, illness, and deaths. My father had cancer, multiple myeloma, and my mother had a heart condition and kidney failure. Both had dialysis. I traveled from Long Island, New York to Newark, New Jersey to help care for them, much of that time in the hospital that I was born in. I will never forget the day that my mother fell at home and was rushed to the hospital. I received a call from her at 2 a.m. "Andy, can you bring my tooth powder to the hospital." Broken arm and severely bruised face and head, all she could think about was what she needed to keep her dentures in place so that she would look good. And, of course I took the 90-minute drive in to Newark at 2:30 a.m., got her tooth powder, came home, and went to work. After all, one good turn deserves another.

A situation involving my father was a little more complicated. Why hadn't the doctor told us, told my father that multiple myeloma is a terminal illness? Why did I have to read about it in a book and then ask him when he planned on telling my father? Why did I have to orchestrate and sit in on the meeting? And then, sometime later, why did I have to make the decision about when to stop dialysis and when to provide the morphine drip and when to increase the morphine? Nothing prepared me for this. There was no one to advise me. Why was I going one-on-one with an oncologist? When he backed off, the staff on the floor, intimidated by the doctor when he was in their presence, provided lots of reinforcement and support once he was absent. "You did the right thing," they would tell me repeatedly. But did I? Later my dad's brother, who I adore, told me the same thing. But did I do the right thing? I still wonder.

CONCLUSION:
REMEMBERING WHAT MIGHT HAVE HELPED

A short-term mutual aid group to help family members like me, in situations that I was in, to deal with the stress of decision-making in this situation might help. To this day I am left with great ambivalence about both my parents' treatment in the hospital. I spoke to one social worker. I thought to myself, "Now we're talking. One of my kind." But not really. It was just more of the same. So, again I'm left with my poetry and what it evokes. I share it here so that it might stimulate your own memories and move you to advocate for short term mutual aid groups for people like me.

Poetry II.

but i have 2 boys

endless corridor
cluttered
white
with
scopes
and
the smell
of the end;

*the curtain opens
to
a bloody ballet:
hoses
and
catheters
and
iv's
and*
   him:

a snarling,
flailing,
spouting,
pulsating
canvas:
      red

each
jab
each
hook:
struggling
with
chemical chains;
and
from
      it all.
so they
found
some
special
cloth and
tethered him
insecurely,
binding
him
in
still
tighter,
refusing
to let
him
go.

the chief
made himself
scarce
so *i* tracked
him
down
and

cornered
him
and
told him:
      "no more."

he shrugged and said:
      "sorry"

and he turned
      away
           from *me*.

before
his
escape
my hand
gripped
him:
twisting
and
jerking
him to
      ATTENTION
only
for him
to hear
once more:
      "no more."

he
bowed his
head
and
turned-
only
more slowly
this time–
and
jangled
the keys

to the prisoner's
      CELL,
proceeding
past the thin
white line.
he stepped through,
seeing what was left of *him*.

and
finally
the chief
left
it
to the glowering
       me,
turning his back
on both of   *us;*
and
disappearing
to
be
seen
       nevermore, nevermore.

and as the
two doors
met
in the middle,
leaving
him
behind

for evermore, evermore:
the
dressed whites
lifted their
heads
and
guided
us
out.

but
not
before
he told an
angel:
      i'm ready to die, but I have two
      boys

and so *he*
kept running
with
us,
for
us,
but
only
until
he
ran
out
of
breath

Poetry III.

cancer

myeloma
my my
myeloma
sigh sigh
myeloma
why why
myeloma
cry cry
my daddy
bye bye

Index

BOOK ORDER FORM!

Order a copy of this book with this form or online at:
http://www.haworthpress.com/store/product.asp?sku=5568

Group Work and Aging:
Issues in Practice, Research, and Education

___ in softbound at $34.95 soft. ISBN-13: 978-0-7890-2881-5 / ISBN-10: 0-7890-2881-6.
___ in hardbound at $59.95 hard. ISBN-13: 978-0-7890-2880-8 / ISBN-10: 0-7890-2880-8.

COST OF BOOKS _____

POSTAGE & HANDLING _____
US: $4.00 for first book & $1.50
    for each additional book
Outside US: $5.00 for first book
    & $2.00 for each additional book.

SUBTOTAL _____

In Canada: add 7% GST. _____

STATE TAX _____
CA, IL, IN, MN, NJ, NY, OH, PA & SD residents
please add appropriate local sales tax.

FINAL TOTAL _____
If paying in Canadian funds, convert
using the current exchange rate,
UNESCO coupons welcome.

❏ BILL ME LATER:
Bill-me option is good on US/Canada/
Mexico orders only; not good to jobbers,
wholesalers, or subscription agencies.

❏ Signature _____

❏ Payment Enclosed: $ _____

❏ PLEASE CHARGE TO MY CREDIT CARD:
❏ Visa ❏ MasterCard ❏ AmEx ❏ Discover
❏ Diner's Club ❏ Eurocard ❏ JCB

Account # _____

Exp Date _____

Signature _____
(Prices in US dollars and subject to change without notice.)

PLEASE PRINT ALL INFORMATION OR ATTACH YOUR BUSINESS CARD
Name
Address
City   State/Province   Zip/Postal Code
Country
Tel   Fax
E-Mail

May we use your e-mail address for confirmations and other types of information? ❏ Yes ❏ No We appreciate receiving
your e-mail address. Haworth would like to e-mail special discount offers to you, as a preferred customer.
We will never share, rent, or exchange your e-mail address. We regard such actions as an invasion of your privacy.

Order from your **local bookstore** or directly from
The Haworth Press, Inc. 10 Alice Street, Binghamton, New York 13904-1580 • USA
Call our toll-free number (1-800-429-6784) / Outside US/Canada: (607) 722-5857
Fax: 1-800-895-0582 / Outside US/Canada: (607) 771-0012
E-mail your order to us: orders@haworthpress.com

For orders outside US and Canada, you may wish to order through your local
sales representative, distributor, or bookseller.
For information, see http://haworthpress.com/distributors

(Discounts are available for individual orders in US and Canada only, not booksellers/distributors.)

Please photocopy this form for your personal use.
www.HaworthPress.com

BOF05